Korean Food Systems

The Republic of Korea (ROK) is projected by 2030 to have the longest living population compared to any nation on Earth. A girl born in the ROK in 2030 will live up to 90.8 years on average. What are the reasons for this improvement in longevity?

Among many insights for longevity among the people of the ROK is the diverse Korean ethnic diet with roots in a traditional diet that has been preserved for centuries. *Korean Food Systems: Secrets of the K-Diet for Healthy Aging* provides an integrated and holistic approach towards the understanding how food systems of the ROK and experiences of the last 60-plus years has been sustained by traditions and ecology integrated with contemporary advances in technology and the economy.

Key Features:

- Discusses the rationale and basis of food systems, traditions of healthy eating, and healthy aging in the Korean population and why by 2030 they will be the longest living population on the planet.
- Reflects on the role of historical, cultural, and traditional food and dietary concepts of Korea and how they have influenced healthy eating habits, contributing to health and longevity.
- Discusses the relevance of the modern genetic concepts of nutrigenomics and epigenetics, metabolic concepts such as circulation, and food concepts such as fermented and functional foods in advancing healthy food concepts and longevity.
- Provides insights on how a large population can advance an integrated holistic food-based approach to longevity and wellness.

As a collaboration between various outstanding authors, the insights from this book can provide global examples to align similar approaches and policies in other countries in different ecologies of planet Earth.

Korean Food Systems

Secrets of the K-Diet for Healthy
Aging

Edited by
Dong-Hwa Shin and Kalidas Shetty

Cover photographs provided by Professor Yoon, Sook Ja.

First edition published 2023
by CRC Press
6000 Broken Sound Parkway NW, Suite 300, Boca Raton, FL 33487-2742

and by CRC Press
4 Park Square, Milton Park, Abingdon, Oxon, OX14 4RN

CRC Press is an imprint of Taylor & Francis Group, LLC

Library of Congress Cataloging-in-Publication Data
Names: Shin, Dong-Hwa, editor. | Shetty, Kalidas, editor.
Title: Korean food systems : secrets of the K-diet for healthy aging / edited by Professor Emeritus Dong-Hwa Shin, PhD, Emeritus Professor of Chonbuk National University, Republic of Korea and Professor Kalidas Shetty, PhD, Professor of Plant Sciences, North Dakota State University, Fargo, ND, US.
Description: First edition. | Boca Raton, FL : CRC Press, 2023. | Includes bibliographical references and index.
Identifiers: LCCN 2022008761 (print) | LCCN 2022008762 (ebook) | ISBN 9781032231129 (hbk) | ISBN 9781032231099 (pbk) | ISBN 9781003275732 (ebk)
Subjects: LCSH: Food--Korea--History. | Diet--Korea. | Longevity--Nutritional aspects--Korea. | Koreans--Nutrition. | Food habits--Korea--History.
Classification: LCC TX360.K6 K65 2023 (print) | LCC TX360.K6 (ebook) | DDC 394.1/2095195--dc23/eng/20220318
LC record available at https://lccn.loc.gov/2022008761
LC ebook record available at https://lccn.loc.gov/2022008762

ISBN: 978-1-032-23112-9 (hbk)
ISBN: 978-1-032-23109-9 (pbk)
ISBN: 978-1-003-27573-2 (ebk)

DOI: 10.1201/9781003275732

Typeset in Caslon
by MPS Limited, Dehradun

Contents

Acknowledgments

Kind acknowledgments to Professor Yoon, Sook Ja for providing the cover photographs

Preface: Perspectives and Vision of the Book

With the advent of human civilization and organized community, humans have always shown the innate desire to live longer and healthier lives. This instinctive desire to live long continues in the modern times from rural to urban living and lifestyles. Overall, the longevity of human life has continued to increase, and life expectancy has continued to grow with the dynamic history of eating, from hunter and gatherer approaches to the changes in the social environment with organization of communities and single-family units. Though longevity has species-specific limits, when animal studies are extended to humans then they show the possibility of living longer than what is currently possible (Lee 2018).

The main factor in the extension of a healthy life is the result of the combination of medical technology that enables the prevention of infectious diseases and the treatment of diseases according to the scientific advances. These advances include the supply of high-quality food as the source of healthy nutrition and personal hygiene through sanitation management. These developments will continue across the world, but the question remains whether the human life span can be extended forever. This is impossible to draw conclusions on right now, based on current scientific advances and developments.

Human life is characterized by natural aging and, ultimately, death. Natural aging is the part of the existing master plan for humanity with earth's ecological limitations and possibilities. Aging, like all animals, has a fixed schedule for a life span based on a species-specific biological clock and can also be affected by day-to-day living and related benefits and challenges of overall physical living (Kontis et al. 2018). Certainly nothing is physically everlasting in this universe as matter is in continuous states of forming and conversion. Even time defined by humans as a mental concept cannot be seen as eternal, and the current universe that is suggested to have been born about 13 to 15 billion years ago is still transforming, and the earth, which occupies one corner of this large space, is predicted to be extinct with a link to the life span of the supporting sun becoming a super nova.

Therefore, taking all insights and evidence we humans understand, the results of insights and studies so far can extend human life as much as possible within the permitted period, but it is not clear whether the limit can be exceeded. Taken together, the results suggest that after 25 to 30 years of age, the body function decreases by 1% every year. Given these predicted phenomena based on current known limits, there is a limit to the length of a disease-free life. However, staying healthy until the end of life can be improved based on our efforts and the processes of these advances can be offered to all humanity to make our dreams of wanting to live longer come true.

It is estimated that the average life span of Stone Age humans was about 30 years old and did not exceed 40 years until modern age. The reason was that early humans were always exposed to the elements of starvation, epidemics, war, and infectious diseases. In Korean folklore, it is mentioned that the well-known Chinese Emperor Qin Shim sent Seobok to various places (including Jeju Island, Korea) and tried to save Bulnocho ("herb for never older" when translated literally), and yet did not escape death for the given limitation of life. In nature, Bristol Pine in the White Mountains of California, USA, has trees that are currently 4,800 years old (Ferguson 1969), which is difficult to compare directly with humans, but many animals live much longer than humans in nature. In 2006, eels in southern Sweden were estimated to have lived for 152 years, and clams caught in Iceland are estimated to be 405 to 410 years old (Das 1994).

The world-renowned longevity zones are the Mediterranean area and Okinawa of Japan. Their longevity has been attributed to their diet and natural environment (Keys 1980; Wilcox et al. 2005). Grandmother Tajima Nabi, the world's oldest 118-year-old who lived in Kagoshima, Japan, was born in 1900 and worked in the field until the 1990s (Kim 2018). The life expectancy of Koreans from the Republic of Korea (ROK) has now increased by 4.5 years every 10 years, starting at 66.5 years in 1980 to 82.4 years in 2016 and is expected to exceed 90 years after 20 years (Lee 2018).

It is reported that a girl born in the ROK in 2030 will live up to 90.8 years on average and, based on this, the ROK is expected to become the longest living country in the world (Chosun Ilbo, 2017.2.25.). Based on this report, the life expectancy is 90.8 years old for women and 84.1 years for men, which is followed by France and Japan. The results were published jointly by the WHO and Imperial College London, UK, and were published in the British Medical Journal, *Lancet* (Kontis, 2018).

Therefore, well before 2030, both men and women of the ROK would likely become the longest living among all people and nations of the earth, surpassing the nations that are currently the longest living, like Japan. According to these estimates, living up to 90 years of age will be very common and, considering individual differences, the probability of healthy living and survival above 100 years of age will also be greatly increased.

Among many reasons for longevity among the citizens of the Republic of Korea is the good Korean diet with lots of food diversity and roots in a traditional diet that has been preserved for centuries. Contemporary citizens of the ROK building from these traditional advantages of food culture have good nutrition, low blood pressure, low smoking rates, and modern access to medical systems when they are young and at critical stages of early life. This contributes substantially to an increased life expectancy that is projected by 2030.

According to the current assessment in the ROK, the average male life span of citizens was over 80 years old in 2015. In the middle of the Joseon Dynasty in 1500–1700, the average life span of males was estimated to be less than 35 years old. Therefore, the life span has been greatly extended over the last 500 years. Now in the modern context it is not just about extending biological life, but about living with good health.

Unlike in the past, where there was high dependence on nature for well-being and life, the current life span extension was primarily determined by the advancement of medical science and technology and the consistent availability and supply of good, quality food. In terms of medical and scientific technologies, personalized precision medical technology, gene therapy, artificial organ replacement technology, tissue engineering, and even traditional medicines and therapies are being developed to prevent or treat certain diseases with new advances and understanding. In addition, food quality has also been advanced using a variety of ingredients to have better taste and balanced nutrition, and cutting-edge processing technology and methods with easy availability in the marketplace. In addition, the additional nutritional improvement approaches have led to the management of supplying the balanced nutrients across all population.

Many advances in science and technology offer other benefits, but the rising costs to enjoy them continue to weigh on consumers. Increasing costs have led to a growing inequality in which expensive new medical technologies and quality foods benefit only certain people who can afford the costs.

This book has been developed with the previously discussed perspectives in mind to provide meaning and guidance on how we will all sustain and manage the quality of a happy life and living. This book was published in the 127th Hallym Round Table Discussion, "Necessary Food and Development Directions for 100 Years of Health," organized by the Korean Academy of Science and Technology, KAST (June 12, 2018). The contents have been rearranged for easy understanding and published in Korean with the title of "Geongang100se jangsusikpumiyagi" by Sikanyeon, the publishing house of the Korea Food Security Research Foundation. I would like to thank KAST and Sikanyeon for their efforts to publicize this important issue to the people. The English edition was made possible by the efforts of Professor Kalidas Shetty, North Dakoda State University, U.S.A., who encouraged the Korean co-authors to translate their chapters into English and edited the English manuscripts by himself. I must thank Sikanyeon for permitting the copyright of the English edition to CRC Press. We hope that this book will help to provide a perspective to protect the health and wellness of not just ROK citizens and society, but lessons can be applied across the world to live a quality and happy life of 100 years of age.

Although longevity is humanity's greatest desire, it is also important to look for the undesired adverse reactions to unsupported longevity with better health and to find the best way to respond effectively with consistent solutions based on science built from long human experiences. Physical weakness due to aging is a natural phenomenon but, according to our approach, it is scientifically possible to maintain good physiological function positively supporting physical and mental wellness and delay aging. Therefore, pre-medical treatment and preventive management of aging are becoming more important, and this book provides some insights from the Republic of Korea experiences.

Finally, on behalf of all the authors of this book, we express our deep gratitude for the continued efforts such as English fine-tuning and sentence rearrangement conducted by Professor Kalidas Shetty, North Dakota State University (NDSU). We would like to express our special thanks to him once again for enhancing the dignity of this book by helping readers understand it in fluent and comfortable expression with a global context.

Dong-Hwa Shin
Emeritus Prof. of Chonbuk National
University, Rep. of Korea

References

Chosun Ilbo, Daily Press (2017) Analysis of expecting life span. Feb. 2. 25.

Das M (1994) Age Determination and Longevity in Fishes. Gerontology 40:70–96.

Ferguson CW (1969) A 7104-Year Annual Tree-Ring Chronology for Bristlecone Pine, *Pinus aristata*, from the White Mountains, California. Tree-Ring Bulletin 29:3–4.

Keys A (1980) Seven Countries: A Multivariate Analysis of Death and Coronary Heart Disease. Cambridge (MA): Harvard University Press.

Kim (2018) Japanese Old Grandpa far Passed Away at 118 years. Seoul, Republic of Korea: Chosun Ilbo (Daily Press).

Kontis V, Bennett JE, Mathers CD, Guangquan Li G, Foreman K and Ezzati M (2018) Future life expectancy in 35 industrialized countries: Projections with a Bayesian model ensemble. Lancet 389(10079):1–7.

Lee (2018) Expecting Life Span. Seoul, Republic of Korea: ChosunIlbo (daily Press).

Willcox B, Willcox C and Suzuki M (2005) The Okinawa Diet Plan: Get Leaner, Live Longer, and Never Feel Hungry. New York (NY): Penguin Random House.

Editors

Dong-Hwa Shin, PhD is an emeritus professor with Chonbuk National University, Jeonju, Korea. He earned a Ph.D in Food Science & Technology from Dongguk University, Seoul, Korea. He has 18 years of experience in the research field at the Food Research Institute in AFDC which is the first Korean government supported food research organization. At this institute he carried out many industry-oriented and applied research projects. After working at the institute, he transferred to Chonbuk National University in the department of Food Science & Technology and served there for 22 years.

During that time, he published 350 research papers, 15 patents, and 23 books. He managed a Regional Research Center (RRC) for supporting food industry in the region, which was fully supported by the Korean government for 10 years. His major field of interest is food fermentation, especially soybean and vegetable-based fermentation. Based on his research, he transferred 30 relevant techniques to related industries to be commercialized. He had served as advisor of different governmental organizations and private food manufacturing companies including CJ and Nongshim, which are the biggest companies in Korea. He was a UNDP/FAO consultant for food industry development at Southeast Asian countries (1983). He is a member of the Korean Academy of Science & Technology (KAST), president of the Korean Society of Food Science

Technology (2002), president of the Korean Society of Food Hygiene and Safety, president of the Korean Association of Food Sanitation (2004–2016) and president of the Food Safety Association. At present he is president of the Korean Council for Sunchang Soybean Fermentation, president of Korea Food Industry Promotion Forum, and is the Director of Shindonghwa Food Research Institute.

Kalidas Shetty, PhD is currently the Associate Vice President for International Partnerships & Collaborations, Founding Director of the Global Institute of Food Security and International Agriculture-GIFSIA, and Professor of Plant Sciences at North Dakota State University, Fargo, USA. Dr. Shetty's research interests focus on the critical role of cellular and metabolic basis of oxygen biology for advancing new innovations in life sciences and especially agricultural and food innovations that advance global food security and health in a sustainable environment.

His specific research interests focus on scientific, educational, and policy strategies to advance climate-resilient health-targeted food security solutions including malnutrition and hunger challenges. In particular, he has developed an innovative "climate-resilient crops for health" research platform to counter diet-linked non communicable chronic diseases (NCD). He has published over 230 manuscripts in peer-reviewed journals and over 50 as invited reviews and in conference proceedings with an H-Index of 75 on Google Scholar.

In 2004, he was selected by the US State Department as the inaugural Jefferson Science Fellow to advise on scientific issues as they relate to international diplomacy and international development. Dr. Shetty has delivered lectures and attended seminars in the areas of Food Biology, Climate Resilient Healthy Food Systems for Food Security & Health and Food Safety in over 50 countries in Asia, Europe, Africa, and the Americas. He also has a deep commitment to global education capacity building.

His current passion is to advance research, education capacity building and policy on "sustainable and ecological basis for climate resilient healthy food systems and food diversity to drive global food security". This vision is based on crops and food diversity, indigenous wisdom, traditional fermentations, and new technology innovations in ethnic and indigenous food systems that incorporate understanding of comparative cellular biochemistry of plant and animal systems and their interactions with microbial systems in diverse ecologies and cultures of earth. This system based integrated model and research platform based on the cellular basis of oxygen biology of food plants and plant-microbial interactions is the basis for new and innovative sustainable agriculture and food solutions to advance climate resilient and health-targeted food security.

Contributors

Soo-Wan Chae
Clinical Trial Center for
  Functional Foods
Jeonbuk National University
  Hospital
Republic of Korea

Hyun Woo Kim
Department of Biotechnology
College of Life Science and
  Biotechnology
Korea University
Seoul, Republic of Korea

Kyong-Chol Kim
Family Physician
Gang Nam Major Clinic
Seoul, Republic of Korea

Sun Min Kim
Department of Biotechnology
College of Life Science and
Biotechnology
Korea University
Seoul, Republic of Korea

Dae Young Kwon
Hoseo University and Korea
  Academy of Science and
  Technology
Republic of Korea

Cherl-Ho Lee
Emeritus Professor
Korea University
Seoul, Republic of Korea

Mee Sook Lee
Emeritus Professor
Hannam University
Republic of Korea

Hyun Jin Park
Department of Biotechnology
College of Life Science and
   Biotechnology
Korea University
Seoul, Republic of Korea

Sang Chul Park
Endowed Chair Professor
Chonnam National University
Republic of Korea

Sea Mi Park
Department of Biotechnology
College of Life Science and
   Biotechnology
Korea University
Seoul, Republic of Korea

Kalidas Shetty
Professor of Plant Sciences
North Dakota State University
Fargo, North Dakota, USA

Dong-Hwa Shin
Emeritus Professor
Chonbuk National University
Republic of Korea

INTRODUCTION

Wisdom and Ecology of Korean Food Systems in the Modern World: Insights and Perspectives on Advancing Diversity of Ethnic Foods for Health and Wellness from K-Diet

DR KALIDAS SHETTY

Professor of Plant Sciences, North Dakota State University, Fargo, USA

Contents

0.1 Introduction

The quality of human life and especially the quality of aging are impacted by the quality of food and associated diet based on the ecology of the food systems, which further has public health consequences. Now with climate change linked to global warming, health-targeted and climate-resilient rationale for advancing global food systems based on food diversity must be aligned to counter the rapid emergence of diet-linked chronic diseases that represent a new challenging reality of global food security (Shetty 2014; Sarkar and Shetty 2014a,b; Sarkar et al. 2020). These global increases in diet-linked non-communicable chronic diseases (NCDs) are resulting in a heavy burden on long-term healthcare management, increasing the costs in aging societies as well as demographically younger emerging

DOI: 10.1201/9781003275732-1

countries, with impacts on the quality of life and national budgets (Shetty 2014). The overall burden of NCDs and associated co-morbidities involves a series of progressive metabolic and cellular malfunctions that manifest in enhancing cellular oxidative stress (i.e., breakdown in respiration-driven oxygen function associated with energy needs) at many cellular and organ levels (Shetty 2014; Shetty and Wahlqvist 2004). This will need NCD countering health-targeted functional ingredient-rich diets designed for the manage-ment of oxidative stress, which can optimize metabolic energy needs to combat NCDs (Shetty 2014; Shetty and Sarkar 2019) with improved impacts on the quality of aging from prevention to delay of these chronic diseases. This suggests that cost-effective strategies of metabolic innovations for NCDs are improved designs of foods from plant, animal and microbial systems based on agroecological diversity with optimized health-targeted impacts on NCDs (Shetty and Wahlqvist 2004; Shetty 2014; Shetty and Sarkar 2019). Improved health-targeted food design must balance both macronutrients and micronutrients but also enrich a wider diversity of other beneficial nutrients and bioactive compounds to counter oxidation-linked mal-functions of NCDs, resulting in better quality of aging and con-tributing to a long life. These health-targeted bioactive-enriched foods are essential to advance healthy community-wide nutrition and quality of life, while concurrently increasing the agroecological diversity (i.e., plant and animal biodiversity) of local food systems with deep-rooted cultural and local ecological influences shaping food choices. These advances will benefit the global society with climate-resilient food systems to manage food production and quality that can impact better health and with impacts on quality aging (Shetty 2014; Shetty and Sarkar 2019).

0.2 Food Diversity Is Essential for Good Health

Food diversity rationale and its relevance to wider resilience must advance the understanding of a sustainable global food and nutri-tional security model. This rationale must be fine-tuned to advance a sustainable and resilient global food production system from a wide diversity of crops and animals in diverse ecologies to meet macro/micronutrient needs along with phytonutrients (e.g., phenolic antioxidants as one example) to counter obesity-linked NCDs (Shetty 2014; Shetty and Sarkar 2019). The NCD burden with substantial impact on co-morbidities also contributes to the failure of the immune response to infections and represents a multi-faceted burden on healthcare systems worldwide, as evident now in the current COVID-19 pandemic. The current food production system and economics associated with it favor a narrow range of food crops with a focus on highly processed, soluble, carbohydrate-enriched foods with low fiber (Shetty 2014; Shetty and Sarkar 2019). These strategies focus on a few cereal crops that are less resilient and not robust in responding to burdens of climate change extremes as they are developed for carbohydrate-based yields rather than inducible responses to abiotic stresses. Abiotic stresses can induce oxidative breakdown, inducing bioactive and nutritional components from the overall carbon flow that can also be a part of healthy human and animal diets.

Unsustainable ecology lacking in food diversity, which leads to narrow and restricted food crop choices and animal foods, is leading to a high consumption of hyper-processed soluble carbohydrates, without micronutrients and oxidative stress protecting phytonutrients. This is contributing to an increasing agroecological imbalance leading to failure of the food systems and is contributing to a NCD co-morbidity burden globally. This health breakdown impact of global food systems requires solutions that are integrated, systems-based strategies with improved and balanced nutrition coupled with health-targeted NCD countering food security that advances human and animal health. Such a strategy also advances sustainable agroecology that is based on crop and food diversity and promoting diverse ethnic food concepts built from all human experiences (Shetty 2014; Sarkar et al. 2020; Shetty and Sarkar 2019).

From a systems-based agroecological rationale, climate-resilient and health-targeted foods, plant, and animal metabolic innovations must be advanced (Shetty and Wahlqvist 2004; Shetty 2014; Sarkar and Shetty 2014b; Shetty and Sarkar 2019). This agroecological-driven metabolic approach has the potential benefit of addressing the quality of primary agricultural production and its impact on food processing challenges while also improving its resilience to climate change. These integrated systems-based agroecological approaches will drive resilient and multi-purpose agricultural systems, supporting more health-targeted and ecologically diverse food systems that better address global food security through crop and food diversity models. These approaches are more resilient with an improved approach to addressing the challenges of human health contributing to the quality of aging (Shetty and Sarkar 2018; Sarkar et al. 2020).

0.3 NCD Co-Morbidities and Post-COVID Implications

NCD co-morbidities from the poor quality of global food systems and lacking in food diversity are key realities facing global food security-linked health challenges (Forouhi and Unwin 2019; Fadnes et al. 2022) and further impacted by the rapid emergence of climate change (Shetty 2014). The current global pandemic is providing early insights on the challenges humanity faces. The COVID-19 pandemic caused by the RNA virus, Coronavirus 2, or SARS-CoV-2, resulted in severe acute respiratory syndrome and further multifaceted metabolic disorders. The rate of infection, mortality, and associated medical complications without specific drugs to target or a vaccine under developmental stages or emergency use approval stages has challenged the wider global community with limited solutions in the early phase of the pandemic. Impacts around the world are diverse, with Europe and the Americas being affected the most with case mortality rates in several countries reaching over 2,000 deaths per million (Corona Virus Resource Center at Johns Hopkins, 2021; Worldmeters Coronovirus Statistics 2021). Meanwhile, across several countries in Asia and Africa and even in countries with food security challenges in the traditional calorie model, low vaccine penetration and poor health infrastructure have mortality rates of 300–1,000 deaths per million (Corona Virus Resource Center at Johns Hopkins, 2021; Worldmeters Coronovirus Statistics 2021), but COVID-19 may have resulted in excess deaths in 2020 and 2021 from all causes indirectly due to overall health infstructure failures. What are the reasons for these differences? Suggested reasons for the differences have been from strict adherence to masks, social distancing, sanitation, rapid testing with app-based monitoring, managed lockdowns and range of still emerging therapeutic support coupled with reduced spread in less dense population zones and rural communities with reduced high calorie diet-linked co-morbidity burdens. It is apparent that susceptibility to COVID-19 infections is far higher in people with co-morbidities linked to NCDs coupled with aging and close living in multi-generational families in urban environments.

Therefore a rationalized and logical basis for integrated health-targeted strategies to explore improved food and nutritional management must be advanced while effective pharmacological and vaccine strategies are being advanced. While current primary critical strategies for prevention and management are effective use of face masks, physical distancing, and sanitization techniques, potential enhancement of overall innate immunity via improved nutritional strategies for both prevention of infection and managing subsequent complications can be part of additional integrated management strategies. Based on epidemiological data across many health challenges, it is established that the quality food and nutrition potentially play a major role in the development of immunity. Important research to pursue is whether there are less incidences of infections in regions of the world with diversity of food with balanced calorie density and potentially have low cases of co-morbidity from lower burdens of diet-linked NCD. This must be explored with more evidence as the potential of improved health and co-morbidity-targeted diet diversity that counter NCDs also have the potential for countering infections by improving overall immunity. However, as we move forward, it is important to understand the chemistry and biochemical functional quality of diverse food systems across ecologies and design health-targeted benefits to communities. Considering the manifestation of clinical symptoms and diverse complications of COVID-19, it is currently very challenging to extrapolate the information or outcome from previous studies. Information needs to be developed for dietary designs for supporting the further validation of infectious disease management outcomes associated with NCD co-morbidities emerging from poor diet with a severe imbalance of macro- or micro-nutrients from failures of the calorie-rich food system. We must build on the success of technologies that have allowed people to conquer hunger and malnutrition in large parts of the world and fine-tune strategies to address new emerging challenges of building climate-resilient and health-targeted food systems based on food diversity across diverse ecologies.

0.4 K-Diet Perspectives and Insights from Korean Food, Culture, and Civilizational Experiences

Korean cultural and civilizational experiences based on the last 70 years in the Republic of Korea (ROK) provide strong insights on how local food diversity and ecological integration helped shape Korean food systems and quality from land and sea. The next eight chapters give a diverse sociocultural and historical journey of the K-Diet, which defines the experience of the ROK since its formation and its advancement to a high-calibre technological society. With the ROK projected to have the longest living population on earth by 2030, it is imperative that we take a close look at how food systems and quality built from a Korean ecology and cultural framework coupled with technological success of the ROK shaped this quality of health, life, and longevity success and what insights the K-Diet and associated diversity of food systems provide to understanding the secrets of this success and longevity. This can provide valuable insights and lessons to other countries globally as it relates to health, wellness, and longevity. This book brings together scientists and technologists from the ROK who have a deep understanding of what has contributed to Korean longevity. Through eight insightful chapters, important clues have been gathered on what has contributed to longevity in the ROK population in the last 70 years that will give rise to the longest living population on earth by 2030. Chapter 1 by Sang-Chul Park provides insights on Korean ethnic foods and provides a new paradigm for healthy longevity. Chapter 2 by Mee-Sook Lee advances further into what has contributed to this longevity by exploring eating insights through what and how the Koreans are and were eating to live long healthy lives. In Chapter 3 by Cherl-Ho Lee, there is an exploration of how Koreans selected food aligned and suitable for their constitution. In Chapter 4, Dae-Young Kwon goes deep into how a traditional Korean diet has contributed to long quality and healthy life. Chapter 5 by Dong-Hwa Shin is focused on Korean fermented foods for healthier longevity. The final three chapters have insights from contemporary times, where in Chapter 6 Kyong-Chol Kim highlights the concepts of how food alters genes with relevance to understanding nutrigenomics and epigenetics and their implications for longevity. Chapter 7 by Soo-Wan Chae highlights that even with a good diet, good blood circulation is vital to our health. And finally Chapter 8 by Hyun-Jin Park provides insights on trends in the health functional food market and highlights how modern food technology and its applications have relevance in advancing healthy foods for healthy living.

References

Corona Virus Resource Center (2021) COVID-19 Map – Johns Hopkins Coronavirus Resource Center (jhu.edu) https://coronavirus.jhu.edu/map.html

Fadnes LT, Økland J-M, Haaland ØA and Johansson, KA (2022) Estimating impact of food choices on life expectancy: A modeling study. PLOS Medicine 19: e1003889, 10.1371/journal.pmed.1003889

Forouhi and Unwin, (2019) Global diet and health: old questions, fresh evidence, and new horizons. Published Online April 3, 2019, 10.1016/S0140-6736(19)30500-8 See Online/Articles 10.1016/S0140-6736(19)3004

Sarkar D and Shetty K (2014a) Diabetes as a Disease of Aging, and the Role of Oxidative Stress. In V Preedy (Ed.). Aging: Oxidative Stress and Dietary Antioxidants. pp. 61–69. Oxford, UK: Elsevier. Chapter 6.

Sarkar D and Shetty K (2014b) Metabolic Mobilization Strategies to Enhance the Use of Plant-Based Dietary Antioxidants for the Management of Type 2 Diabetes. In V Preedy (Ed.). Aging: Oxidative Stress and Dietary Antioxidants. pp. 289–296. Oxford, UK: Elsevier, Chapter 27.

Sarkar D, Walker-Swaney J and Shetty K (2020) Food diversity and in-digenous food systems to combat diet-linked chronic diseases. Current Developments in Nutrition 4 (Supplement 1):3–11, (10.1093/cdn/nzz099).

Sarkar D and Shetty K (2014) Metabolic stimulation of plant phenolics for food preservation and health. Annual Review of Food Science and Technology 5:395–413.

Shetty K (2014) Systems Solutions to Global Food Security Challenges to Advance Human Health and Global Environment Based on Diverse Food Ecology. Pages 65–73. A policy position paper presented at the conference on Food Safety, Security and Defense: Focus on Food and the Environment, convened by the Institute on Science for Global Policy (ISGP), on October 5–8, 2014 at Cornell University, Ithaca, New York, U.S. (ISBN: 978-0-9861007-0-3).

Shetty K and Sarkar D (2018) *Editorial:* Advancing ethnic foods in diverse global ecologies through systems-based solutions is essential to global food security and climate resilience-integrated human health benefits. Journal of Ethnic Foods 5:1–3. (10.1016/j.jef.2018.02.003)

Shetty K and Sarkar D (2019) Introduction: Metabolic-Driven Ecological Rationale to Advance Biotechnological Approaches for Functional

Foods. In: Food Biotechnology Series, Shetty K and Sarkar D (Ed.). Functional Foods and Biotechnology: Sources of Functional Foods and Ingredients. pp. 1–4. Boca Raton, USA: CRC Press (Taylor and Francis Group), Chapter 1.

Shetty K and Wahlqvist ML (2004) A model for the role of proline-linked pentose phosphate pathway in phenolic phytochemical biosynthesis and mechanism of action for human health and environmental applications. Asia Pacific Journal Clinical Nutrition 13:1–24.

Worldmeters Coronovirus Statistics (2021) https://www.worldometers.info/coronavirus/

1

KOREAN ETHNIC FOOD PROVIDES A NEW PARADIGM FOR HEALTHY LONGEVITY

Endowed Chair Professor, Chonnam
National University

Contents

1.1 Introduction

The first official record in human history on the search for elixirs to overcome mortality is the *Gilgamesh Epic*, written 5,000 years ago in clay plates with cuneiform letters, found at ancient remains of Uruk in the Mesopotamian region. The first hero of humanity, *Gilgamesh*, wished to save the life of his best friend, *Enkidu*. He went down to the bottom of the sea for the Plant of Heartbeat (*sham-mu an-nu-u sham-mu ni-kit-ti*) to resurrect his friend. Though he succeeded in acquiring it, the elixir was unhappily stolen by a serpent (George 2003). Since this *Gilgamesh* legend, a multitude of myths on elixirs pursuing immortality have been popular all around the world. Greek mythology illustrates the divine foods for immortality as ambrosia and nectars. Chinese mythology indicates peaches offer immortality (仙桃, 蟠桃). Indian mythology claims amrita and soma provide immortality, even with an intake of smallest portion. Most of these mythic elixirs are of plant origin in the form of vegetables or fruits as juice, fermented drinks, mixture, or the fruit body itself. These legendary elixirs emphasized something edible, symbolizing the mystic value in special foods (Park 2019).

After the mythic legendary times, the mystery search period began, when the official historic record on longevity pursuit was enforced by the first Chinese emperor, *Qinshi-huang* (秦始皇). Although in vain, the governmental and systematic trials to acquire the elixirs of life opened a new era of longevity pursuit. But the failure of reckless geographic expeditions for elixirs to the legendary places prompted a shift to the direction to develop the artificial technology of alchemy instead of finding the natural elixirs. The alchemy for elixirs had been flourishing in China, Arabia, and later Christian societies up to the 17th century. In this period, the imaginary fountain of youth, holy grails, and philosopher's stone or special pills composed of jade, cinnabar, or hematite have been prepared, albeit in vain. With emergence of the mechanism-based logic period, the concept and enthusiasm for immortality pursuit had been criticized to be rejected by the scientific disputes on safety and efficacy of these approaches. Since then, the ancient mysteries and even fraudulent explanations on human life span extension have been discarded, but the human desire to live long has not been abandoned (Park 2019).

1.2 Calorie Restricted Diets for Longevity

Among many approaches and techniques for life span extension, the current trend in food and dietary pattern for human longevity will be briefly described in this chapter. So many varying fad diets being pursued for human longevity have confused people and, as a result, have come and gone, like ebb and tide, such as low-carbohydrate diet, low-calorie diet, high-protein diet, low-fat diet, balanced diet, and Atkins diet. Therefore, in this chapter, it is more appropriate to concentrate only on the ethnic or ethnic perspective focused diets, which are not specifically targeting some diseases or special condition effects but rather targeting the general overall heathy improvements for longevity.

To provide context to the main tenants of this chapter, the recent trend of calorie restriction should be mentioned. The most popular dietary trend for longevity pursuit is based on calorie restriction (CR), which has been proposed by many disciplines. This was first publicly suggested by Alvise Cornaro in his books about the secrets to live long and well with measure and sobriety (Scheafer 2005). His book *Discorsidella vita sobria*, describing his regimen of CR, was extremely successful, and influenced the European community strongly to change the concept of aging by rejecting conventional wisdom that old age was a period of misery and decay. Since his books on CR and sober life, celebrities started following his suggestions, including Benjamin Franklin. Not only in Western society, but also in the East, CR has been acknowledged traditionally as one of the best ways to live long by many of the religions, including Buddhism, Taoism, and Hinduism. Taoists had been thinking and practicing more strongly about the efficacy of lifestyle and influences on longevity not only by physical but also by mental and spiritual health. Some Taoist diets called for *bigu* (辟穀, avoiding grains) to achieve immortality. Taoists often encouraged practitioners to be vegetarians to minimize harm (Symonds 2007). The taoist tradition of avoiding grains has incessantly influenced the oriental culture. Recently, with scientific investigations, the value of CR has been emphasized and evidence has been emerging with a variety of protocols using many different animal models (Park 2019).

Moreover, the tremendous increase in diseases of affluence in modern civilization has led the public to understand that many diseases were caused by changes in diet. Therefore, the Paleolithic (paleo) diet of our ancestral caveman has been proposed as a natural approach to be a good substitute diet to the modern calorie-rich diets. The paleo diet is mainly based on foods, available to Paleolithic humans, including vegetables, fruits, nuts, roots, and meat and excluding foods such as dairy products, grains, sugar, legumes, processed oils, salt, and alcohol or coffee. The paleo diet, with a recommendation of fewer processed foods and less sugar and salt, is consistent with the present mainstream advice of diet in general. Theory-wise, the evolutionary discordance hypothesis indicates that many chronic diseases and degenerative conditions evident in modern Western populations could have arisen because of a mismatch between stone age genes and recently adopted lifestyles. Advocates of the paleo diet argue that modern people should follow a diet that is nutritionally closer to that of their Paleolithic ancestors (Zuk 2013).

Another interesting suggestion for healthy diet is a macrobiotic where the goal is to balance the yin and yang elements of food; this means that grains are a staple, supplemented with other foods such as vegetables and soy, and certain kinds of cookware should be avoided. Hufeland, who coined the word macrobiotics in the context of food and health, considered macrobiotics as a science, aimed at prolonging and perfecting life as a medical philosophy on a higher level than the curative, preventative, or health levels of medicine (Lerman 2010). These patterns of diet for better health, mainly based on restriction principle, have been emphasized by the elites, which influenced the contemporary people to adopt the principle as one of the behavioral correction strategies for longevity.

However, the practical inconvenience and difficulty in pursuing restricted diets in daily life limited their application. Nevertheless, the recent criticism of CR for its limited effects only for the caged animals but not for the free, open field–living ones has weakened its value. Furthermore, criticisms by nutritionists of the paleo diet and macrobiotic diet for their limited nutritional balance also have restricted their wide application.

1.3 Conflicts of Diets in Longevity Pursuit

For the pursuit of longevity, it was presumed necessary to eat something ambrosia-like, nectar-like, or amrita-like in the ancient period, for which legendary searches for elixirs had been actively pursued. However, the revolutionary concept of restriction principle then started to prevail recently, resulting in restraining the search for elixirs of longevity. This dichotomy of eating something or not to eat much in general has confused and frustrated those who look to food for health and longevity. Generally, food scientists are apt to recommend specific foods with quantity for health maintenance and disease prevention, while many nutritionists are prone to restrict the foods and to emphasize quality and balance rather than quantity. This conflict of quality versus quantity remains as a centuries-old longstanding philosophical debate of what is more relevant. Therefore, it was natural that the concept of optimization of foods was raised by Buttriss (Buttriss 2000), who defined the optimal diet as the diet that maximizes both health and longevity through preventing nutritional deficiencies as well as reducing risks of diet-related chronic diseases by balancing intakes of nutrients and their quality. Nonetheless, the current trend of food processing and engineering industries is practically targeting several major goals for healthy food products. The approaches include glycemic index, low fat to right fat, heart health, well-being (digestive support, detoxification, enhancement of mental wellbeing, energy, immune system, and skin health), individualization (personalized, daily dosing, age appropriate), and functional foods (chemoprevention, prevention of allergy, osteoporosis, and menopausal syndrome) as some examples. These issues are closely associated with production and consumption of food for the promotion of health. Consequently, the tremendous amount of industrial food marketing for advancing health has led people to feel confused and uncertain.

1.4 New Paradigm of Longevity Food, Based on Ethnic Food

Despite various foods being listed as longevity foods, the criticisms have continued on these issues due to lack of scientific evidence, practical difficulty of wide availability, and potential side effects. Therefore, it might be pertinent to define longevity food in terms of practical and tangible aspects. For this purpose, in this chapter, I have proposed a new definition of longevity food as *the traditional ethnic food in long-living population zones with scientific evidence for promoting health*. The reason for the special emphasis on long-living population zones is that it considers lifestyle and dietary behavior of the relatively higher number of people who live long in that specific zone, which would ensure their own ethnic foods for health and longevity. Their longstanding experiences and records of mortality would confirm the efficacy of the regional food for health and longevity than any other theoretical or conceptually introduced diets without a basis of their own ecology. But the practical questions remain and these are: Is the nature of the traditional ethnic foods in a long-living population zone different from other similar areas or is there something extraordinary in their area? Are the lifelong dietary habits of long-lived people different from ordinary people? Is there scientific evidence that the ethnic foods or dietary behaviors are linked to longevity?

Based on these questions, several key discoveries in the field of human longevity effects of foods have been discovered and better defined. The first case is the Mediterranean diet, where the concept was first publicized to reflect the food patterns typical of Greece and southern Italy by Ancel and Margaret Keys (Keys and Keys 1975). After accumulation of epidemiological data mainly from the Seven Countries Study, the diet has profoundly influenced the nutrition society and its related medical and industrial affiliations and collaborations (Keys 1970, 1980). The primary aspect of this diet includes a proportionally high consumption of olive oil, legumes, unrefined cereals, fruits, and vegetables; moderate to high consumption of fish; moderate consumption of dairy products (mostly as cheese and yogurt); moderate wine consumption; and low consumption of non-fish meat and non-fish meat products. The impressive impact of the Mediterranean diet has been derived from what is considered as a paradox concept from the point of view of mainstream nutrition, which suggests that regardless of a relatively high consumption of oily food, people living in Mediterranean countries have far lower rates of cardiovascular diseases than in countries such as the USA; this is named the Mediterranean Paradox. A parallel phenomenon of less cardiovascular diseases by wine consumption is known as the French Paradox. If not supported by epidemiological data for the ethnic foods of the Mediterranean area in terms of higher longevity, the efficacy of the diet would not have been readily accepted. The second case is the discovery of the Inuit's secret of their ethnic diet. Dyerberg discovered haphazardly that the peculiar pattern of diseases and dietary habits of the Inuit in Greenland are closely linked. He observed that coronary heart disease in the Inuit population is a rarity, which led him to pay special attention to their food consumption, of which the diet included high protein, low carbohydrates, and high fat, essentially of mammalian marine origin. Compared with Danish food, the fatty acid pattern of the consumed lipids showed a higher content of long-chain polyunsaturated fatty acids. Describing the serum cholesterol level as a function of the nutritional fatty acids, the presence of a lower serum cholesterol level found in the Greenland Inuit was not explained by conventional logic; therefore, he proposed a special metabolic effect and relevance of the long-chain polyunsaturated fatty acids from marine mammals. And this discovery has opened a new field of omega 3/6 fatty acids ratio for management of cardiovascular disease and other related health effects (Bang et al. 1971, 1976; Dyerberg et al. 1977). The contrast between the Mediterranean diet and Inuit diet is the emphasis on different fatty acids; monounsaturated fatty acids, especially of oleic acid in the Mediterranean diet and polyunsaturated fatty acids in the Inuit ethnic food. Discovery of this positive effect of the unsaturated fatty acids toward better health facilitated new products from food industries and in human nutrition. The third case is the Okinawan ethnic diet. People from the Ryukyu Islands that are part of Okinawa prefecture in Japan have the highest life expectancy in the world. The traditional diet of the islanders contains 30% green and yellow vegetables, with small quantities of rice (instead, the staple is the purple-fleshed Okinawan sweet potato), small quantity of fish, and more soy and other legumes. Specifically, pork is highly valued in Okinawa with a unique cooking process of steaming or boiling without sizzling or roasting. The islanders are noted for their low mortality from cardiovascular disease and certain types of cancers, compared by age-adjusted mortality of Okinawans versus Americans, illustrating that an average Okinawan was 8 times less likely to die from coronary heart disease, 7 times less likely to die from prostate cancer, and 6.5 times less likely to die from breast cancer than an average American of the same age. The Okinawan ethnic food confirms the value of food of plant origin, cooking process, and calorie restriction as well (Willcox et al. 2005, 2007).

1.5 Korean Ethnic Food as a New Elixir for Longevity

Through a survey of Korean centenarians on a variety of life behaviors and dietary patterns, the uniqueness of Korean ethnic food could be unveiled. The initial main questions on the Korean ethnic foods that have been assessed for longevity foods are as follows: 1) What are the regional area factors for the difference in traditional foods between long-living population zones and ordinary areas? 2) What are the lifelong time factors for the difference in dietary behaviors between a long-living population zone and ordinary area?

3) What can be the scientific evidence for contribution of those foods or dietary behaviors to longevity? To answer these questions, several issues of food and dietary patterns of Korean centenarians in the long-living population zone have been assessed.

1. The first issue of food resources

Meals of centenarians were primarily focused on plant foods such as cereals, legumes, and their products, vegetables, fruits, and so on. The average intake of cereals was mostly derived from rice as a staple food. They consumed vegetables with a large portion of vegetable intake in forms of various blanched types (*Namul*) (Lee et al. 2005). They also consumed soybean-fermented foods, such as *Doenjang* (miso equivalent), *Chungkukjang* (natto equivalent), *Gochujang* (pepper paste), or *Ganjang* (soybean sauce) (Kim et al. 2016). Fruit intake was very low, compared to vegetable intake. They consumed animal foods, including meat, poultry, and eggs; fish and shellfish; and dairy products in limited amounts. When assessed by the criteria for a well-balanced diet, which specify a dietary diversity score of >3.0 and a dietary variety score of >18.0, 91.9% of these individuals scored above 3.0 in the dietary diversity score and 48.7% scored above 18.0 in the dietary variety score (Shin and Jeong 2015; Park et al. 2008). These data indicated that the traditional foods consumed by centenarians are enriched with a variety of food types with good balance and a spectrum of functional qualities such as anti-mutagenic, anti-oxidative, anti-carcinogenic, lipid lowering, peroxide scavenging, and immune enhancing potentials (Kimm and Park 1982; Lee et al. 2001; Park 1996; Park et al. 1996; Park and Lee 2002). Although the consumption of fruits was lower than expected, those fruit functional qualities can be compensated by higher vegetable consumption. Therefore, it can be summarized that the combination of a variety of food resources with multiple health-protecting effects in Korean ethnic food can contribute to improved health conditions of the people who consume them.

2. The second issue of the cooking process

When the cooking process of the Korean ethnic food was analyzed, several unique patterns could be observed. The first is the blanching of vegetables for eating rather than fresh state. The blanching can reduce the nitrate content of the vegetables and can eliminate the toxic contaminants effectively. Furthermore, through blanching, the vegetables shrink, which facilitates their quantitative consumption, leading to higher utilization of fibers. The second aspect is the boiling of meats. Both beef and pork were mainly boiled or steamed for consumption rather than roasted or sizzled. This cooking process of meat would reduce the fat content, facilitate detoxification, and prevent the formation of mutagens, since the formation of meat pyrolysis-based toxic by-products can be blocked (Lee et al. 1987, 1988). The other Korean favorite cooking process is pan frying. This pan-frying process for vegetables, fish, and meat with sesame oil or perilla oil makes it more edible, detoxifies, and prevents the formation of mutagens. Furthermore, the traditional style of a combination of vegetables and meat together to eat would be healthy and safe because this combination may contribute towards the suppression of activation of mutagens during metabolism (Park 2008). Therefore, it can be suggested that the Korean traditional methods for cooking by blanching, boiling, and pan frying would be the most effective cooking methods to prevent the formation of mutagens during the cooking process, which would surely contribute to the reduction of the most aggressive cancers and other degenerative diseases.

3. The third issue of nutritional compensation by fermentation

When Korean ethnic foods were analyzed, the dominant consumption of plant origin food raised a warning on the possible nutritional deficiency of vitamin B12, which is mainly derived from animal food or dairy products. However, the prevalence of vitamin B12 deficiency in Korean centenarians was not higher when compared to cohorts in Western nations. It was a big mystery that Korean centenarians are nutritionally well balanced for vitamin B12 and without deficiency despite their vegetable-oriented dietary habits. And it was observed that Korean centenarians have consumed soybean fermented foods such as *Doenjang, Chungkukjang, Gochujang,* and fermented vegetables such as kimchi daily as well as seaweed frequently throughout their lives. And it was amazing to discover that these fermented vegetables and seaweed have eventually proven to be the efficient sources for vitamin B12 (Kwak et al. 2007, 2010, 2012). Therefore, it can be proposed that the Korean traditional ethnic foods can compensate for the nutritional deficiency of vegetable foods by the fermentation process, which would overcome the unbalanced food composition for the health of long-living people consuming a Korean diet.

4. The fourth issue of restriction versus optimum

Male centenarians consumed 85.9% of the estimated energy requirement (EER) for men aged 75 years, 2,000 kcal/d, and female centenarians consumed 77.9% of EER for women aged 75 years, 1,600 kcal/d. The observed percentage of EER for energy intake in both Korean male and female centenarians was much higher when compared to the 60% found in a study of Okinawan centenarians (Park et al. 2008). Along with the higher energy intake, male centenarians consumed more proteins and carbohydrates than female centenarians. However, fat intake was not different (Shin and Jeong 2015). From these data, it can be summarized that the traditional dietary pattern of Korean centenarians indicates the optimum consumption of calories rather than restriction, which would ensure the physically active lifestyle of long-living people.

5. The fifth issue of life beyond food conditions

It is obviously beyond debate that the food factor would not be solely responsible for human longevity. In addition, the time periodicity of food intake, gathering of family to dine, and sharing of the foods with neighbors are the traditional dietary patterns of Koreans, which would contribute to the healthiness of the Korean ethnic food. Furthermore, the gender and environmental effects could be illustrated by the observation that the male centenarians in the mountain zone have better health than the female centenarians in the flat zone (Park et al. 2008). Therefore, Park's Temple Model of Longevity has been previously proposed that natural, social, and behavioral variables would work cooperatively and collectively to support longevity (Park 2013). The food factor is only one of the behavioral variables, which include nutrition, exercise, relationships, and participation. However, there is no doubt that the food factor is one of the most appealing and relevant conditions for human longevity. Furthermore, gene to food and food to environment interactions should be taken into consideration for in-depth analysis, which implies that the human longevity should be understood in collective terms of space and time of life (Kim et al. 2016, Park 2013). Therefore, the significance of ethnic food with a long history of practical applications and scientific evidence cannot be overstated for further application and understanding of human longevity from studies on food effects on human health.

Conclusion

Ethnic foods sufficiently support the basic spatial and temporal conditions for human longevity from food and guarantee the longstanding safety and efficacy for the people who have consumed it from the lived local ecology and food diversity. Many ethnic foods have been suggested to be effective and good for health and longevity, from which much scientific evidence for health has emerged. Extending this rationale, Korean ethnic food can be evaluated for its value as a longevity-supporting food. In summary, the essence of Korean ethnic food can be characterized as having a balance of nutrients, based on a combination of diversified food resources, the nutritional compensation by fermentation, and the safe ways of cooking for minimizing toxicants and preventing the formation of a health hazard in cooked foods as well as healthy dietary habits. Taken together, it would be reasonable and timely to conclude that Korean ethnic food can be included in the list of global longevity foods for its health-promoting quality, based on scientific evidence and longstanding experience of being built from local ecology and food diversity.

Acknowledgments

The main concept of this manuscript has been published in the *Journal of Ethnic Food* (Park 2016). The author deeply appreciates all the members of the Korean Centenarian Study of Seoul National University and Chonnam National University, and special thanks to Dr. Lee MS, Dr. Kwak CS, and Dr. Oh SI for their devotion and enthusiasm in food and dietary pattern study of centenarians.

References

Bang HO, Dyerberg J and Nielsen AB (1971) Plasma lipid and lipoprotein pattern in Greenlandic West-coast Eskimos. *Lancet* 1:1143–1145.

Bang HO, Dyerberg J and Hjøorne N (1976). The composition of food con-
    sumed by Greenland Eskimos. *Acta Medica Scandinavica* 200:69–73.
Buttriss J (2000) Nutrients requirements and optimization of intakes. *British
    Medical Bulletin* 2000(56):18–33.
Dyerberg J, Bang HO and Hjorne N (1977) Plasma cholesterol concentration
    in Caucasian Danes and Greenland West-coast Eskimos. *Danish
    Medical Bulletin* 24:52–55.
George A (2003) *The Babylonian Gilgamesh Epic, introduction, critical edition
    and cuneiform texts*, Vol. 2. Oxford (UK): Oxford University Press.
Keys A (1970) Coronary heart disease in seven countries. *Circulation*
    41:I1–211.
Keys A (1980) *Seven countries: a multivariate analysis of death and coronary
    heart disease*. Cambridge (MA): Harvard University Press.
Keys A and Keys M (1975) *How to eat well and stay well the Mediterranean
    way*. Rome (Italy): FAO.
Kim SH, Kim MS, Lee MS, Park YS, Lee HJ, Kang SA, Lee HS, Lee KE,
    Yanh HJ, Kim MJ, Lee YE and Kwon DY (2016) Korean diet:
    Characteristics and historical background. *The Journal of Ethnic Foods*
    3:26–31.
Kimm SW and Park SC (1982) Evidence for the existence of antimutagenic
    factors in edible plants. *Korean Journal of Biochemistry* 14:47–59.
Kwak CS, Lee MS and Park SC (2007) High antioxidant properties of
    chungkookjang,a fermented soybean paste, may be due to increased
    aglycone   and   malonylglycoside   isoflavone   during   fermentation.
    Nutrition Research 27:719–727.
Kwak CS, Park SC and Song KY (2012) Doenjang, a fermented soybean
    paste, decreased visceral fat accumulation and adipocyte size in rats fed
    with high fat diet more effectively than nonfermented soybeans. *Journal
    of Medicinal Food* 15:1–9.
Kwak CS, Lee MS, Lee HJ, Whang JY and Park SC (2010) Dietary source of
    vitamin B12 intake and vitamin B12 status in female elderly Koreans
    aged 85 and older living in rural area. *Nutrition Research and Practice*
    4:229–234.
Lerman RH (2010) The macrobiotic diet in chronic disease. *Nutrition in
    Clinical Practice* 25:621–626.
Lee MS, Mo SM, Kim JH and Park SC (1988) Mutagenicity of pyrolytic
    products of Korean animal protein foods by Salmonella typhimurium-
    microsome test. 2. Mutagenicity of varying customary cooked meats.
    Environ Mut Carcinogen 8:105–125.
Lee MS, Mo SM and Park SC (1987) Mutagenicity of pyrolytic products of
    Korean animal protein foods by Salmonella/mammalian-microsome
    test. *Enivron Mut Carcinogen* 7:85–102.
Lee MS, Woo MK, Kwak CS, Oh SI and Park SC (2001) Analysis of tra-
    ditional Korean food patterns based on the database of favorite Korean
    foods. *Annals of the New York Academy of Sciences* 928:348–352.

Lee MS, Yeo EJ, Kwak CS, Kim KT, Choi YH, Kwon IS, Kim CH and Park SC (2005) Gender difference in health and nutritional status of Korean centenarians. *Journal of Korean Gerontological* 15:65–75.

Park SC (1996) *Intervention of carcinogenesis and aging process.* Seoul (Korea): APCRI, Seoul National University Press.

Park SC (2008) Diet and longevity: a lesson from Korean centenarians. *Healthcare Restaurant* 2:56–59.

Park SC (2013) Comprehensive approach and outcome of Korean centenarian studies. In: Suh SJ and Choi HK editors. *Aging in Korea; today and tomorrow.* 3rd ed. pp. 290–303. Seoul (Korea): Federation of Korean Gerontological Societies.

Park SC (2016) Ethnic food for longevity pursuit: assessment of Korean ethnic food. *The Journal of Ethnic Foods* 3:167–170.

Park SC (2019) *Magnum Opus 2.0.* Seoul: UDeumJi Press.

Park SC and Lee MS (2002) Database for Korean ethnic food: essential condition for nutritional genomics and functional nutrigenomics. *Food Sci Ind* 35:43–50.

Park SC, Lee MS, Kwon IS and Kwak CS (2008) Environment and gender influence on the nutritional and health status of Korean centenarians. *The Asian Journal of Gerontology and Geriatrics* 3:8–16.

Park SC, Lee MS and Oh SI (1996) Present status of domestic research on screening for antimutagenic, anticarcinogenic and antioxidative components in Korean ethnic foods. *Journal of Korean Association of Cancer Prevention* 1:46–51.

Scheafer D (2005) Aging, longevity, and diet: historical remarks on calorie intake reduction. *Gerontology* 51:126–130.

Shin DH and Jeong DY (2015) Korean traditional fermented soybean products: Jang. *The Journal of Ethnic Foods* 2:2–7.

Symonds M (2007) *Tai Chi Diet: food for life.* London (UK): Life Force Publishing.

Willcox B, Willcox C and Suzuki M (2005) *The Okinawa Diet Plan: get leaner, live longer, and never feel hungry.* New York (NY): Penguin Random House.

Willcox BJ, Willcox DC, Todoriki H, Fujiyoshi A, Yano K, He Q, Curb JD and Suzuki M (2007) Caloric restriction, the traditional Okinawan diet and healthy aging. The diet of the world's longest-lived people and its potential impact on morbidity and life span. *Annals of the New York Academy of Sciences* 1114:434–455.

Zuk M (2013) *Paleo fantasy: What evolution really tells us about sex, diet, and how we live.* New York (NY): WW Norton & Co.

2

KOREAN LONG LIVING PEOPLE: WHAT AND HOW TO EAT TO LIVE

MEE SOOK LEE

Emeritus Professor of Hannam University

Contents

Human life expectancy has increased substantially due to worldwide industrial development and major advances in medicine with an overall improvement of nutritional status. This has particularly impacted South Korea, which has the fastest-growing aging population in the world, with more than 14% of the elderly population above the age of 65. This is much more rapid in 2022 predicted by the National Statistical Office in 2001. South Korea has reported that in the 2016 Census of Population and Housing (KOSIS 2017) report that the population aged 65 or older surpassed the youth population under the age of 15. The number of elderly aged 60 or older was be higher than the number of children under 5 in 2020, and overall 22% of the world's population will be over 60 by 2050 (WHO 2018). Likewise, in the world including S. Korea, the average life expectancy (expected life expectancy) has increased rapidly along with the increase in the elderly population, which is nearing the age of 100 (Figure 2.1).

However, many elderly citizens now live 8 to 10 years of their later life with very poor quality of life due to chronic diseases, poor mental

DOI: 10.1201/9781003275732-3

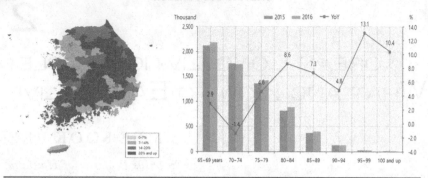

Figure 2.1 Increasing the elderly population; the ratio of elderly aged 65 years or older by city or county and the rate of population increase by age of elderly.

Source: KOSIS (2017), 2016 Population and Housing Census.

health, and inadequate diet. This is not a desirable phenomenon, so it is time to think deeply and act and practice from the perspective of "healthy aging." A community of nations have called on the World Health Organization (WHO 2018) to advance consultation and guidelines to develop and maintain functional capabilities that enable well-being of the elderly population. Although "elderly" generally indicate and show the challenges of mental and physical problems such as bent bodies, inability to move themselves, chronic diseases, and dementia, the condition of the longevity is so diverse that some elderly people are as healthy and engaged in social activities as young people, which reflects healthy aging. Therefore, we need to look at how the elderly live and find a way towards a higher quality of "healthy aging."

Health is an evolving process of healthy living that highly depends on a good quality diet that has been practiced by communities in a their own ecologies and among other things also important is genetics, medical benefits, social activities, and exercise. Many studies have shown that genetic factors are some of the important longevity factors, but only 25% of the good health and longevity (WHO 2018) are associated with genetic factors. More important are environmental factors such as living conditions, mental and physical activities, lifestyle, and quality dietary factors. Among the environmental factors, the most influential factors for health care are quality and diversity of diet and with lifestyle. Many studies of healthy, long-lived centenarians focused on the

S. Korean population, which has significant merit for developing good insights for guidelines (Mee Sook Lee 2002: Seoul National University's Institute of Physical Science and Aging, The Chosun Ilbo (2003)) to improve the unhealthy eating habits that have been followed can be overcome by finding indicators of proper healthy food intake and healthy eating behaviors; from such deeper insights take the right path to "healthy aging."

2.1 Health Status of Long Living People

Looking at the medical health of the centenarians, the average value of hematological parameters such as levels of blood glucose, glycosylated hemoglobin, cholesterol, triglycerides, albumin, and vitamin B12 were all within a normal range. Unlike older people in their 60s and 70s, there was a unique range: Those who had the disease had very low rates of high blood glucose (diabetes), hypertension, hypercholesterolemia and hyperlipidemia, and no patients had hepatitis B (Table 2.1).

The prevalence rate of chronic disease of centenarians is significantly lower than that of those aged 70 or older. According to the 2016 statistics on chronic diseases released by the Korea Centers for Disease Control and Prevention in 2017, the prevalence rate of those aged 70 or older with reported conditions were diabetes (16.4% for men, 29.0% for women), hypertension (64.2% for men, 72.5% for

Table 2.1 Hematologic parameters of Korean centenarians

PARAMETER (UNIT)	AVERAGE VALUES	PERCENT OF ABNORMAL
Blood glucose (mg/dl)	106.2 ± 24.7	8
Hemoglobin (g/dl)	11.7 ± 1.4	10
Hematocrit (%)	35.4 ± 3.9	14
Total cholesterol (mg/dl)	164.3 ± 35.2	18
HDL-cholesterol (mg/dl)	41.8 ± 10.6	32
LDL-cholesterol (mg/dl)	110.1 ± 30.3	22
Triglyceride (mg/dl)	98.6 ± 53.9	2
Ca (mg/dl)	8.96 ± 0.44	0
Albumin (g/dl)	3.75 ± 0.39	20
Vitamin B12 (pg/ml)	428.9 ± 217.7	0
Folate (ng/ml)	5.99 ± 3.82	26
Hepatitis B (antigen)	—	0

women), hypercholesterolemia (16.4% for men, 29.0% for women), and hepatitis B (2.7% for men, 1.7% for women).

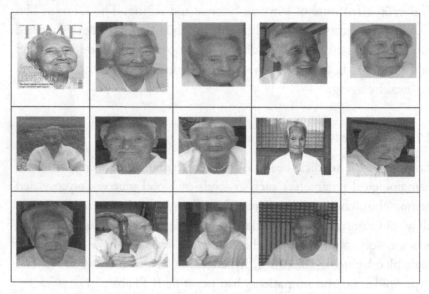

For centenarians, the low incidence of diabetes, arteriosclerosis, or hypertension is a common phenomenon not only found in South Korea but also in Japan and Italy. As already known, high blood glucose, high blood pressure, high cholesterol level, and hyperlipidemia are the main causes of death from chronic diseases such as cardiovascular disease, diabetes, and hypertension, so these desirable hematological indicators of the centenarian may explain the health longevity of the centenarians.

Also, the centenarians had no hepatitis B carriers due to good liver condition, and all of the blood albumin levels indicating protein nutritional status were good except for centenarians who were not able to move well. Hemoglobin and hematocrit level in the blood were also good, so there was little anemia. In foreign countries, there is a high incidence of vitamin B12 deficiency in older people, which causes various diseases in the nervous system and cardiovascular system. However, in Korea, centenarians were eating plant foods such as grains and vegetables that have little vitamin B12 but the level of vitamin B12 in their blood was good. This was found to be supplemented by *Doenjang* (soybean paste), *Ganjang* (soy sauce) and other sauces, and *Kimchi* and seaweed, although they eat less animal food.

As such, Korean centenarians, unlike those in their 70s and 80s, have lived a healthy, long life by avoiding various degenerative diseases such as hypertension, diabetes, and cardiovascular disease. Therefore, we should pay attention to their healthy lifestyle and eating habits to find out how the centenarians who lived in an era where they did not receive some medical care were able to avoid the deadly diseases.

2.2 Healthy Lifestyle of Long Living People

When investigators in S. Korea linked to this chapter visited a centenarian's home without notice, most of the female centenarians were doing housework such as gardening, scrubbing, washing clothes, and chopping red peppers, while the male centenarians were doing farmwork such as cutting grass in the fields and rice paddies. Surprisingly, some male centenarians went to the real estate office every day, some people often went out to town for teatime, went to do banking, and some female centenarians visited the homes of their children living in the same neighborhood every day, and went to the community center. Therefore, it is thought that it is essential to find out what kind of lifestyle the centenarians have and what kind of healthy lifestyle has made them physically and mentally healthy, and to practice it as well.

Most healthy centenarians were able to effectively function in their daily lives without the help of others, such as washing their face, brushing their teeth, using toilets, eating, walking, dressing and bathing, and also cognitive functions were healthy for their age. They also have a high confidence and positive attitude about their health, with about 70% of centenarians thinking they are healthy. This positivity and confidence in health is due to the lack of chronic diseases such as diabetes and hypertension and while also living healthy and busy daily lives such as housework, gardening, farming, and going to the neighborhood. Furthermore, it is thought that they could have been able to maintain good health by continuing their physical activities, such as farming and housework.

Low rates of centenarian smoking and drinking alcohol than those of the elderly aged 65 or older may also have been an important factor in maintaining their good health. Because Korean centenarians lived through difficult times, most people (over 80%) did not have dentures, but they did not have much inconvenience in eating food overall and were consuming a normal diet from their local ecology and based on availability. Few people took special supplements, health foods, and nutritional supplements. In addition, unlike the old saying that older people get less sleep, the centenarians had enough sleep for 8 to 10 hours. Information indicates that they had good sleep, supporting their healthy mind and body because they were doing proper physical activities such as housework and gardening that defined their daily good purpose.

2.3 Food and Dishes That Long Living People Like

Today, the S. Korean society largely has a wide variety of choices of abundant and delicious and wholesome foods. There are many private and governmental programs to introduce delicious and healthy foods that are pleasant to the eyes and mouth, including advertisements showing videos of eating many delicious foods at once, and promoting healthy foods that are good for the body. In addition, many people take pictures before eating food and send it to acquaintances and therefore it has become part of social engagements through new medias.

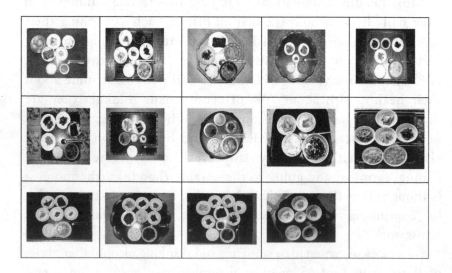

Yet even in the presence of such abundance and choices the incidence of chronic diseases such as diabetes, hypertension, cardiovascular disease, and cancer are rising sharply, and it is not clear which of these foods we eat that contributes to living a healthy and long life. Could we find the key to solving this question in the meals of the centenarians? So, what and how did the centenarians eat, so that they lived a healthy, long life? These are very important questions for understanding the secrets for healthy long life.

The important bottom line is that after looking into the diet of the centenarians, there is no particular food or healthy food that Korean centenarians enjoy. However, it was a diversified balanced diet consisting of rice, soup, and side dishes, typical of a traditional Korean diet, and a vegetable-based meal that often consumed a variety of *Namuls* (blanched vegetables) rather than raw vegetables, sauces such as *Doenjang* (soybean paste), and *Gochujang* (red pepper paste) (Table 2.2).

Going deeper into further analysis, starting first with nutrient intake status, the question is: If centenarians and the elderly are eating a similar Korean traditional diet, then what is the difference between them and the current elderly above 65?

According to the current nutrition status of the elderly in Korea, there is a general lack of balanced nutrition, except for the problem of calorie-burdened overnutrition found in some urban classes (1.2% of people aged 65 and over). According to the 2017 Korea National Health and Nutrition Examination Survey (KNHANES VII-2) (Ministry of Health and Welfare · Korea Centers for Disease & Prevention 2017), 40.2% of the elderly aged 70 or older were under

Table 2.2 Diet patterns of Korean centenarians

1. *Rice (Bap)*
2. *Kimchi:* Fermented mixture of vegetables and spices (mainly garlic, ginger, hot pepper) with salted small fishes
3. *Namuls:* Blanched and seasoned vegetables
4. *Doenjang soup: Doenjang* (soybean paste) with vegetables or tofu

Vegetable food-oriented diet
- **Variety of vegetables**
- **Fermented foods: *Doenjang*, kimchi**

75% of the estimated energy requirement (EER). In addition, the average percentage of people who ate less than the estimated average requirement (EAR) was 47.1% protein, 86.5% calcium, 82.9% vitamin A, 20.6% thiamin, 70.2% riboflavin, 65.5% niacin, and 57.5% vitamin C, indicating that the elderly were not eating well. In particular, the lack of nutrition intake is more severe in rural areas and low-income elderly than in urban areas (Mee Sook Lee 2001).

The results of comparing the nutrition status of centenarians with that of Korean recommended dietary allowances (RDA) of those over 75 years of age are shown in Table 2.3. Although it is difficult to compare with intake due to the lack of RDA of 100-year-old people, the Index of Nutrition Quality (INQ: The quantity of a nutrient per 1,000 kcal in a diet comparing to the RDA of a nutrient) showed that all nutrients except calcium and riboflavin were very good at over 0.75 (75%). Overall, calcium and riboflavin are the most limited nutrients among S. Korea's 75-year-olds and older population. Comparing this, we can conclude that centenarians have a much lower proportion of the undernourishment than those aged 75 or older.

Table 2.3 Energy/nutrient intake of Korean centenarians

ENERGY/NUTRIENT (UNIT)	INTAKE *	PERCENT OF RDA*	INDEX OF NUTRITION QUALITY (INQ) **
Energy (Kcal)	1318.0 ± 425.5	80.9 ± 24.7	
Protein (g)	45.7 ± 20.8	75.8 ± 35.0	0.90 ± 0.26
Fat (g)	21.1 ± 12.2	–	–
Carbohydrate (g)	240.0 ± 77.5	–	–
Fiber (g)	5.0 ± 3.0	–	–
Ca (mg)	494.3 ± 416.3	70.6 ± 59.5	0.73 ± 0.53
P (mg)	689.0 ± 289.9	98.4 ± 41.4	1.20 ± 0.30
Fe (mg)	8.78 ± 5.01	73.2 ± 41.7	0.79 ± 0.32
Vitamin A (µg RE)	653.8 ± 516.8	93.4 ± 73.8	1.08 ± 0.74
Vitamin B_1 (mg)	0.79 ± 0.43	79.3 ± 42.7	0.92 ± 0.28
Vitamin B_2 (mg)	0.64 ± 0.39	53.6 ± 32.4	0.67 ± 0.34
Niacin (mg)	9.46 ± 4.53	72.9 ± 34.9	0.86 ± 0.27
Vitamin C (mg)	71.70 ± 47.97	128.4 ± 84.3	1.25 ± 0.70

*Intake and percent of RDA: mean ± standard deviation/RDA (recommended dietary allowance) for age 75 or older Koreans.
**Index of Nutrition Quality: The quantity of a nutrient per 1,000 kcal in a diet compared to the RDA of a nutrient.

Even though centenarians eat an ordinary Korean traditional diet just like the average elderly, the better nutrition status is thought to be the result of differences in dietary pattern and dietary composition, or overall dietary food diversity. This leads to the interesting path to determine the type of diet centenarians prefer, what kind of food choices they like and make, and what kind of food or dishes they dislike.

After analyzing the dietary patterns of the centenarians, they preferred the dietary patterns of "*Bap* (rice) + Soup (or *Jigae*) + Side dishes" (Figure 2.2). Generally, a diet consisting of "*bap*, soup and side dishes" increase the diversity of foods consumed, rather than "*Bap* + Soup" or "*Bap* + Side dish" or "One-dish meal" and this then had a desirable benefit on better nutrition.

The centenarians preferred *bap* (rice) as their main food, and they disliked porridge and western soup (Figure 2.3). Among soup and

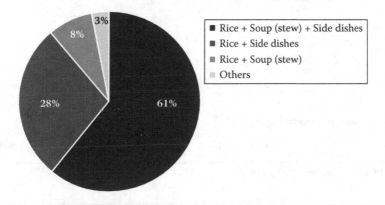

Figure 2.2 Menu patterns.

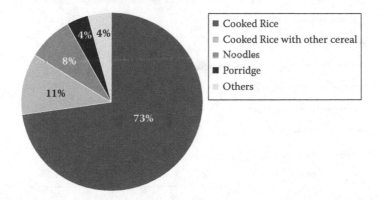

Figure 2.3 Patterns of staple foods.

Jigae (stew) the most frequent intake was that of *Doenjang soup* (soybean paste soup) with vegetables or tofu, *Doenjang jigae* (soybean paste stew) or *Gochujang jigae* (red pepper paste stew) (Figure 2.4). Kimchi, which always goes as a side dish, with most frequent use of cabbage-kimchi and radish leaf-kimchi. The other side dishes other than kimchi consumed the most was *Namuls* (blanched and seasoned vegetables) and seasoned vegetables. The next type of side dish was the consumption of *Jangs* (sauces) such as *Doenjang* (soybean paste), *Gochujang* (red pepper paste), and *Ssamjang* (assorted *jangs* and seasoned vegetables, seasoning), but the consumption rate of raw vegetables was very low (Figure 2.5).

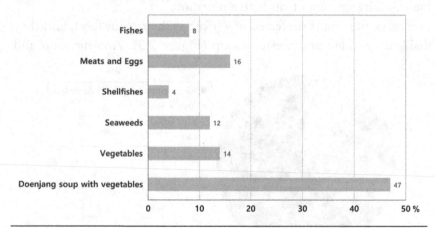

Figure 2.4   Patterns of soup and stew.

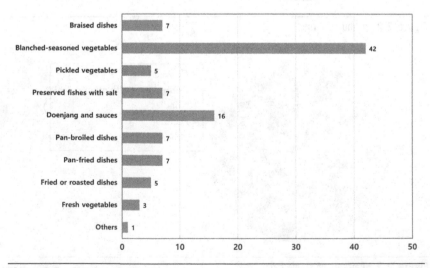

Figure 2.5   Patterns of side dishes.

As shown in their picture of a typical meal, most of the centenarians always consumed *bap* (rice), *kimchi, namuls,* pre-stored side dishes made of vegetables grown in the garden or nearby areas, and soup or *jigae* made of *jangs* such as *doenjang* (soybean paste) and *gochujang* (red pepper paste). They also frequently consumed seaweed such as laver or sea mustard. The results of asking centenarians about their favorite food groups and their likes and dislikes of specific foods are shown in Table 2.4. There was no specific food group that was disliked too much, thus allowing flexibility. Overall, their favorite food groups were vegetables, beans, and seaweed, the same as on their picture of a meal, followed by fruits, mushrooms, and fish. Centenarians' favorite dishes were rice, starch and pancakes, *namuls,* rice cakes, potatoes and sweet potatoes, followed by soup, grilled dishes, and stir-fried dishes. Among the dishes they disliked to some degrees were salted vegetables, porridge or western soup, salted fish, and fried foods, as these foods were salty or oily and swallowed without chewing. In addition, considering that 45% of people always consumed *jangs* such as *doenjang, ssamjang,*

Table 2.4 Favorite foods and dishes of Korean centenarians

FAVORITE FOOD GROUPS (%)	
Vegetables	96.8
Legumes	90.5
Seaweeds	88.9
Fruits	79.4
Mushrooms	79.4
Fishes	73.0
Eggs	68.2
Meats	63.5

LIKED DISH (%)		DISLIKED DISH (%)	
Cooked rice	98.4	Pickled vegetables with salt	55.6
Pan-fried dishes	95.2	Porridge or western soup	46.0
Braised dishes	95.2	Preserved fishes with salt	42.9
Namuls (Blanched-seasoned vegetables)	93.7	Fried dishes	41.3
Rice cakes	93.7		
Potato, sweet potato	90.5		
Soups or stews	87.3		
Grilled or baked dishes	87.3		
Stir-fried dishes	85.7		

gochujang, and soy sauce, the fermented soy foods in Korea, this may have helped the overall health of the Korean centenarians.

In summary, the Korean centenarians meal consists of *bap* (rice), *kimchi, namuls,* and *doenjang soup* (soybean paste soup), and are a typical longevity diet.

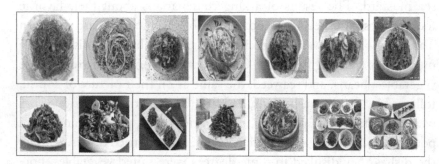

In particular, close attention must be given to the meals of the Korean centenarians that are part of the Korean traditional diet that has protected their healthy longevity on par in relevance as the Mediterranean diet or Okinawa diet, which are well-known longevity diets for those specific ecologies and communities. As shown in Table 2.5, the Korean traditional diet consists of different combinations of the Mediterranean diet with a diversity of combinations increasing the potential healthy outcome and longevity.

The big difference is that a Mediterranean diet is a more animal food-oriented diet and a Korean traditional diet is a more vegetable food-oriented diet. Moreover, the Mediterranean diet has consumption of wine, fruit, and raw vegetables, and the Korean traditional diet

Table 2.5 Contrasting dietary patterns between Mediterranean diet and Korean traditional diet

<MEDITERRANEAN DIET>	<KOREAN TRADITIONAL DIET>
Fresh vegetables	Blanched vegetables (Namuls)
Wine	Rice wine (Maggeoli), Soju
Feta cheese, yogurt	Doenjang (soybean paste),Gochujang (hot pepper sauce)
Fruits	Vegetables
Marine fishes or mollusks	Seaweed
Fresh food products	Fermentation products
Animal foods	Vegetable foods

has rice wine, and vegetables consumed as *namuls* (blanched vege-tables) and not raw. In common are that the ingredients are different, but fermented foods are preferred. The commonality between an Okinawan diet and Korean traditional diet is that they are vegetable food-oriented diets, and the methods for boiling meat are similar. On the other hand, the kinds of vegetables used are different, and unlike the Okinawa, which mainly uses fish for its consumption of omega-3 fatty acids, the Korean diet has perilla oil and perilla seeds along with fish. There is also the difference between eating *Sungnyung* (scorched-rice water) and mineral water instead of drinking green tea, which is common in Okinawa. As such, the longevity diet might be relying more on diversity and mixing, cooking process, and fermented foods that have been eaten in the specific ecology of the community for a longer time than any specific food.

2.4 How Do Long Living People Eat?

Centenarians and the elderly eat the same traditional Korean diet, so why do centenarians live a long life and not other people above 65 years? They are eating a vegetable-oriented meal consisting of rice, *kimchi*, vegetables, and *doenjang*, some of which are healthy, and others are not. It is essential to look at what differences have emerged from the dietary habits in modern times rather than the dietary pattern. In other words, what type of food or what food you eat is important, but also how you eat, namely, eating habits or eating behaviors, are also important factors, and these were examined in the diet habits of the centenarians (Table 2.6).

The most distinctive feature of the centenarians' dietary habits is eating three meals. One of the centenarians said he was eating two meals because it had become a habit since he was young, and the mealtimes were always the same. Such regular eating habits contrast with those of modern times. In modern times, skipping breakfast for various reasons combined with irregular eating habits such as eating late or having a late-night snack without having lunch or dinner on time is observed. Would the centenarians' regular eating of three meals drive their regular lifestyle and enables their healthy longevity? As already known, eating habits, especially those who wake up late in the morning and skip breakfast, this can not only

Table 2.6 Dietary habits of Korean centenarians (%)

Meals per day (number/day)	2 times	7.9	Preference of Taste	Sweet food	Like	93.6
	3 times	92.1			Dislike	4.8
Regularity of mealtime	Regular	100.0			So-so	1.6
	Irregular	0.0		Salty food	Like	65.1
Speed of eating a meal (min.)	≤15	17.7			Dislike	28.6
	15~20	40.3			So-so	6.3
	>20	41.9		Hot food	Like	52.4
Appetite	Good	94.4			Dislike	41.3
	Bad	5.6			So-so	6.3
Meals with family	Yes	64.8		Fried food	Like	37.1
	No	35.2			Dislike	53.2
					So-so	9.7

reduce the efficiency of their work, but can also lead to bulimia where eating more food in other meals follows, increasing a bad diet and health risks.

Also, centenarians typically eat an optimum portion size of diverse foods each time. These are typically the same amounts for breakfast, lunch, and dinner, thereby maintaining a constant intake. This would be logical and fits well with the lifestyle of getting up early and going to sleep early. If they had a snack for lunch or afternoon, they reduced the amount of food for the next meal. It is already a well-known fact that a repeated burden on the stomach with eating and overeating or binge eating just like in the modern lifestyle, is harmful to health.

This shows that by making a habit of eating a certain amount of regular meals at a given time, your body will be able to turn into a healthy body that can eat as much as it needs. Therefore, this will be a more effective way to protect your health than any herbal tonics or nutritional supplements.

The favorite food group among the dietary habits of the centenarians shows that most food groups are not specifically preferred but eaten as a combination of diversity of foods and therefore bring consistent diversity in health benefits for a healthy metabolism. The most disliked food, the *Zhangachi* (pickled vegetables with salt), was about 55%, and these were consumed less than the other combinations of preferred foods. In general, there is no large choice of specific food eaten in large amounts. In terms of the taste of the dishes, it turned out that they liked sweets and but not oily and greasy ones, which was like the overall combination of favorite food groups. Although they liked sweets, the high percentage eats fiber-rich carbohydrates (grain), not simple sugars, and also the high intake of abundant fiber through vegetables and moderate balanced total calories seemed to have helped them avoid chronic diseases such as diabetes and hypertension.

The ratio of people who like salt is also quite high because they are used to salty-tasting foods such as *kimchi* or *Doenjang* (soybean paste), but considering that the percentage of people who dislike much higher salty food than *kimchi* was also high. Centenarians who like spicy foods were almost equal at 50-50 with those who disliked them, and greasy types were more disliked. In addition, the higher diversity of foods generally consumed (the number of foods taken) likely contributed to the more balanced and good nutrition for healthy longevity. Therefore, when comparing the centenarians with the dietary variety score (DVS), which is used as one of the diet quality assessment methods, the DVS was higher, i.e., the number of foods consumed (variety) was higher, contributing to a much better intake of nutrients than the other narrow combinations (Table 2.7). This shows that, even if you are a healthy person, eating a wide variety of food (diversity) is important for lifelong

Table 2.7 Energy/nutrient intake of Korean centenarians by DVS group

		DVS (DIET VARIETY SCORE)		P VALUE
		HIGH	LOW	
Percent of RDA †	Energy	88.9 ± 27.3 ‡	75.3 ± 21.2	0.0303*
	Protein	88.8 ± 39.4	61.7 ± 25.2	0.0019**
	Ca	73.5 ± 38.9	44.1 ± 34.6	0.0025**
	P	113.4 ± 42.6	84.6 ± 36.1	0.0054**
	Fe	79.1 ± 41.2	53.6 ± 30.9	0.0075**
	Vitamin A	111.6 ± 79.3	71.5 ± 62.4	0.0297*
	Thiamin	88.6 ± 48.7	65.9 ± 26.4	0.0250*
	Riboflavin	67.4 ± 37.6	45.3 ± 28.4	0.0109*
	Niacin	82.9 ± 35.3	60.7 ± 30.7	0.0101*

Notes
† RDA (recommended dietary allowance) for age 75 or older Korean people.
‡ Intake and percent of RDA: mean ± standard deviation.

Table 2.8 Dietary habits of Korean nonagenarians (%)

Meals per day (number/day)	2 times	6	Pleasure of mealtime	Yes	85.7
	3 times	94		No	14.3
Regularity of meal Time	Regular	95.8	Regular activity	Yes	72.6
	Irregular	4.2		No	27.4
Meals with family	Yes	80.4	Drug daily	Yes	31.7
	No	19.6		No	68.3
Appetite	Good	85.7	Symptoms of disease (number)	0	51.8
	Bad	14.3		≥1	48.2

health, contributing to longevity. Another interesting food-related habit among Korean centenarians is that they eat with their family, which likely contributes to a high total food score and better nutritional status. Therefore, eating with their family or neighbors can be an important factor in their health.

In addition to the survey of 168 centenarians, others who are aged 90 or older were also surveyed and show similar results (Table 2.8). Therefore, we should emulate the good dietary habits of centenarians for healthy longevity.

These desirable eating habits, such as eating a diversity of foods, reducing the number of salty foods and greasy or fried foods, and, if possible, eating with your family will be important keys to good health, potentially contributing to longevity.

The last important aspect in the dietary habits of the centenarians is that they eat in proportion to their activity. We know already that calorie restriction (CR) is necessary for prolonging life and eating in proportion to activity needs supports CR.

However, after studying the centenarians, there was no strict and absolute CR. Overall, as a normal part of the decline in activity due to age, they are eating less than they were when they were young, but there was no CR as defined by current research for modern context. Healthy centenarians working on farms such as field farming, grass planting, and gardening were eating more than 2,000 kilocalories with the addition of a snack meal when there was a lot of farming. When there was no hard farmwork, they did not snack and returned to their usual diverse diet. The average calorie intake of the rural Korean centenarians was about 1,700 kcal for men and about 1,250 kcal for women. According to the energy requirement formula by DLWT (doubly labeled water technique), (TEE = $\alpha-\beta \times$ age (yr) + PA [$\gamma \times$ Wt (kg) + $\delta \times$ Ht (m)], a white European man is required to have 1,545 kcal/day, and a woman needs 1,173 kcal/day. In comparison, healthy centenarians in Korea were not having small meals (calorie restriction) but eating a moderate amount of food according to their activity. In other words, the healthy centenarians regularly ate a certain amount of food and increased or decreased the amount of food they ate according to their activity. This suggests that, it is more important not to overeat or binge eat than the calorie restriction but eat according to activity needs.

Therefore, in order to live healthy contributing to longevity, one must develop desirable dietary habits: A regular diet of three meals (at a fixed time), eating a variety of foods, avoiding salty or greasy food, and a diet that meets the amount of activity without overeating or binge eating.

2.5 The Excellence of Korean Traditional Diets

Below are perspectives on the scientific basis for the excellence of Korean traditional diets, which protected the health of the centenarians.

First of all, the diet of centenarians who ate Korean traditional diets satisfied the dietary guidelines (to prevent chronic diseases such as cancer) suggested jointly by the American Cancer Society and other academic societies. All the diversity of foods consumed turned out to be suitable except for the high intake of salt, as shown in Table 2.9. This shows that Korean centenarians' diet has allowed them to live a healthy and long life without getting chronic diseases. In addition, compared to the Okinawan food pyramid (Table 2.9), which is recommended for a healthy, long life, there was no shortage of key nutrients, except for a small shortage of calcium intake due to the low consumption of dairy products. Therefore, one can suggest that one can live a healthy, long life with Korean traditional diets.

It is known that the characteristic of Korean traditional diets enjoyed by Korean centenarians is a vegetable-oriented diet. In addition, they use various vegetables such as *kimchi* and *namuls*, and use *doenjang* and other fermented soy foods. Thus, if the scientific evidence proves that these foods have healthy functions such as

Table 2.9 A comparison between Korean centenarian's diets and the eating guidelines for health in foreign countries

GUIDELINES		SATISFIED	KOREAN CENTENARIAN'S DIETS
USA Unified Dietary Guidelines (* Suggested by American Cancer Society, American Heart Association, American Dietetic Association, American Institutes of Health)	1. Eat a variety of foods, mainly from plant sources	O	DVS (Diet Variety Score) 17.2 Plant source 83.4%
	2. Eat at least 5 servings of vegetables and fruits daily	O	Vegetables 220 g/day Fruits 80 g/day
	3. Eat at least 6 servings of grain-based foods daily	O	Grains 220 g/day (mainly, rice)
	4. Make complex carbohydrates the basis of the diet (more than 55% of total calories)	O	Carbohydrate 70.3% of total kcal (mainly, grains)
	5. Limit fat intake to 30% or less of total calories	O	Fat 14.4% of total kcal
	6. Limit total salt intake to less than 6 g per day	×	Salt 10–12 g/day
Okinawa Food Pyramid	1. Eat 10 vegetables and fruits daily (9–17 servings)	O	Plant-based diet: Vegetables 220 g/day Fruits 80 g/day
	2. Eat 10 whole grains daily (7–13 servings)	△	Grains 220 g/day (but, mainly polished rice)
	3. Eat 3 calcium foods daily (2–4 servings)	×	Dairy foods 40 g/day, Ca intake 355 mg/day
	4. Eat 3 flavonoid foods daily	O	Legumes 30 g/day Soybean-fermented food 17 g/day Vegetables 220g/day
	5. Eat 2 omega-3 fatty acids daily (1–3 servings)	O	Perilla seed & oil Fish (mackerel, pacific saury)
	6. Drink fresh water and tea daily	△	Fresh or boiled water, no tea
	7. Drink alcohol in moderation or not at all	O	Drinking, often: Male 16.7%, Female 22.9%

anti-cancer, antioxidant, and anti-aging effects, such functions that can prevent chronic diseases such as cancer, cardiovascular disease, and diabetes, then the Korean traditional diet could be called a healthy longevity diet.

Because vegetables are free from saturated fats and have high fiber content, this is implicated in reducing blood cholesterol levels and not allowing spikes in blood glucose level and therefore contributing to the prevention of cardiovascular disease or diabetes. Moreover, it also contains various phytochemicals, which potentially have anti-oxidant, anti-cancer, and anti-aging effects. It is therefore essential to determine and confirm whether the vegetables that centenarians are enjoying are effective in preventing chronic diseases such as cancer, cardiovascular disease, and diabetes. Towards this purpose and goal, the anti-mutagenic, antioxidative, lipid peroxide reduction, and immune-enhancing potential benefits of common vegetables popular among Korean people was evaluated. Table 2.10 to Table 2.12, Figure 2.6, and Figure 2.7 (Oh and Lee 2003) were examples of research results.

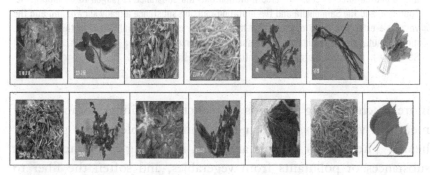

As such, most of the favorite commercial common vegetables are rich in bioactive ingredients that act as anti-mutagenic, antioxidant, lipid peroxide scavenging, anti-cancer, and immune stimulating foods. Therefore, the Korean traditional diet is supports a longevity diet.

In addition, one of the characteristics of Okinawa's longevity diet is a cooking method of stewing pork and not frying or grilling, which potentially reduces carcinogens. Similarly, in traditional Korean cooking methods that are also helpful for healthy longevity, frying and grilling is absent. In traditional Korean cooking, vegetables are blanched for *namuls* or put into soup rather than consumed as raw vegetables. The meat is boiled in water rather than grilling or roasting and, further, meat or fish are cooked with various vegetables, and vegetable oils such as sesame oil and perilla oil are used

Table 2.10　Anti-mutagenic potentials of some vegetables by Ames test †

VEGETABLES	TA98(−)	TA100(−)	TA98(+)	TA100(+)
Mustard leaves	+3 *	0	0	2
Korean lettuce	3	0	2	2
Chard	3	0	0	0
Perilla leaves	4	0	4	4
Shepherd's purse	3	1	4	4
Pumpkin	1	0	0	1
Korean wild chive	2	2	0	0
Sedum	3	0	2	3
Wild water dropwort	2	4	4	4
Garlic	1	4	2	3

* Inhibition rate; 0: <10%, +1: 10~25%, +2: 25~50%, +3: 50~75%, +4: >75%.
† Antimutagenicy test method developed by Ames: Salmonella typimurium TA98 and TA100 is added and cultured to cause reverse mutation and the substance is judged to be mutagenic. Therefore, add the Salmonella and the mutation-causing substance already known, and add the vegetable extract to it to measure how much reverse mutation is inhibited. In this case, the indirect mutagenic potential can be measured by adding S9mix (+), a liver extract, and without S9 mix (−), the direct mutagenic potential can be tested.

more. Such cooking methods as blanching, boiling, combining of meat and vegetables, and stir-frying in vegetable oil are good for health. The reasons for this are: first, blanching can remove toxic substances or pollutants from vegetables, and soften the fiber to help with digestive absorption and therefore more nutrient is bioavailable than raw vegetables. Therefore, even if there is a slight loss of water-soluble vitamins, it is a good cooking method for high intake of fiber or vitamins overall and low intake of toxic substances. *Namuls*, a characteristic side dish of the Korean diet does not have additional calorie-rich dressing, but only a little sesame oil and sesame seeds, unlike western salads. Therefore, it is a very good healthy recipe that can contribute a lot of fiber and vitamins with fewer calories. Second, types of soup such as *doenjang soup, jigae*, and *tang* (stew), which are characteristic of Korean meal patterns, do not produce carcinogens because the cooking temperature is not high, and because vegetables are cooked with meat or fish, which prevents the generation or formation of carcinogens in food. It is already well known that heating animal products at 150°C or higher

Table 2.11 Lipid peroxide scavenging potentials of Korean some vegetables

VEGETABLES	INHIBITION RATE ON LIPID PEROXIDATION (0~1 mg/Assay)	SCAVENGING EFFECT OF DPPH RADICAL † (0~0.5 mg/Assay)	INHIBITION RATE ON THE MDA-BSA CONJUGATION ‡ (0~100 mg/Assay)
Carrot	0 *	2	3
Mustard leaves	2	2	4
Korean lettuce	2	2	4
Chard	2	2	4
Perilla leaves	2	2	4
Shepherd's purse	3	3	3
Pumpkin	2	2	3
Wild chive	2	1	3
Sedum	3	3	3
Wild water dropwort	3	4	3
Garlic	0	2	4
Buckwheat	3	2	4
Korean radish	0	1	3

* Inhibition rate; 0: <10%, +1: 10~25%, +2: 25~50%, +3: 50~75%, +4: >75%.
† DPPH radical scavenging effect: Free radical reacts indiscriminately with several molecules in the cell, damaging cells and tissues. To see how effectively the experimental material reduces these radicals, a method to measure how much reduce a certain amount of free radicals using DPPH (α,α-diphenyl-β-picrylhydrazyl) a stable free radical reagent.
‡ MDA-BSA conjugation inhibitory effect: Malondialdehyde (MDA) combines directly with biomolecules (proteins) in cells to cause protein deformation, cell membrane destruction, mutations, etc. Therefore, a method to measure how much the experimental substance inhibits the conjugation with malondialdehyde (MDA) and bovine serum albumin (BSA).

produces a lot of carcinogens, so stir-frying or boiling at low temperatures can be beneficial to health rather than high temperatures such as frying, grilling, or barbecuing (Mee Sook Lee 1992). However, making the soup too salty is bad for health, so keeping it bland or using low salt is preferred. Third, the use of vegetable oils such as soybean oil, sesame oil, and perilla oil rather than animal oil is beneficial, as these oils can contribute to prevention of cardiovascular disease. In particular, the high use of perilla seeds and perilla oil rich in omega-3 fatty acids is a very different characteristic compared to other countries.

Table 2.12 Anti-cancer effects of some vegetables on the cancer cell lines (IC 50)

VEGETABLES	SNU-638[†]	MCF-7	HELA
Perilla leaves	40.59	91.27	79.84
Radish leaves	39.3	320.61	232.05
Carrot	65.56	2472.75	778.72
Mustard leaves	554.92	290.46	141.52
Sedum	600.22	162.43	319.75
Chives	250.59	164.1	53.43
Chard	133.02	112.23	112.38
Mugwort	107.26	303.21	115.12
Korean zucchini	–	482.74	570.39
Korean radish	–	∞	∞
Pumpkin	–	10742.01	∞
Cabbage	–	∞	∞
Sea fusiformis	53.42	49.87	45.55
Sea lettuce	83.74	48.32	48.21
Onion	–	2822.88	126.51

[†] Names of cancer cell line: SNU-638 (human stomach cancer cell line), MCF-7 (breast cancer cell line), HeLa (cervical cancer cell line).

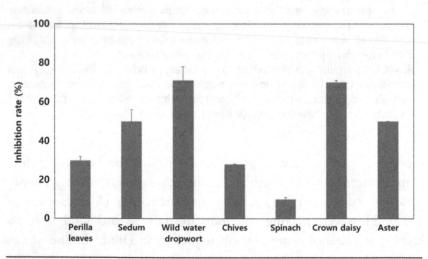

Figure 2.6 Scavenging effects of DPPH radical by some vegetables.

As such, it would be advisable to learn the Korean traditional diet and stay healthy like Korean centenarians; using the cooking methods of a Korean traditional diet are good for preventing chronic diseases such as cancer and cardiovascular diseases.

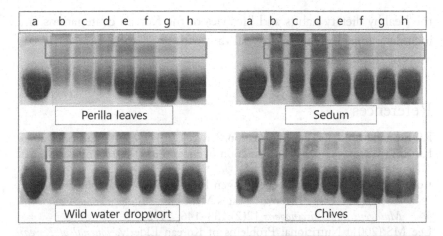

Figure 2.7 Inhibition rate of water fraction of some vegetables on the conjugated MDA with BSA.

Notes

a: BSA (100 μℓ) + PBS (900 μℓ), b: BSA (100 μℓ) + MDA (100 μℓ) + PBS (800 μℓ), c: BSA (100 μℓ) + MDA (100 μℓ) + sample (12.5 μℓ) + PBS (787.5 μℓ), d: BSA (100 μℓ) + MDA (100 μℓ) + sample (25 μℓ) + PBS (775 μℓ), e: BSA (100 μℓ) + MDA (100 μℓ) + sample (50 μℓ) + PBS (750 μℓ), f: BSA (100 μℓ) + MDA (100 μℓ) + sample (100 μℓ) + PBS (700 μℓ), g: BSA (100 μℓ) + MDA (100 μℓ) + sample (200 μℓ) + PBS (600 μℓ), h: BSA (100 μℓ) + MDA (100 μℓ) + sample (400 μℓ) + PBS (400 μℓ).

Conclusion

Korean centenarians, who have lived healthy, long lives similar to people in other well-known healthy diet ecologies such as Mediterranean and Okinawan communities, were eating a Korean traditional diet consisting of "*Bap* (rice) + Soup + Side dishes," which have several layers of health benefits contributing to longevity. The soup consumed was mainly *Doenjang* soup (soybean paste soup), and for side dishes, it consisted of basic *Kimchi* and various *Namuls* and/or other small amounts of animal side dishes combined with vegetables and boiled and blanched with low heat with no toxic side effects. They also ate three regular meals, adjusted the amount of meals according to the activity, and had a diet where they did not overeat but rather had small meals as required for activity. They also ate a wide variety of foods (food diversity) evenly and ate less foods that were salty or oily. Along with these, they restrained themselves from drinking and smoking, engaged in diligent physical activities through everyday life, and lived well with their neighbors. Therefore, one can benefit from the keys to healthy aging by following the healthy dietary habits and lifestyles of the Korean centenarians and include a good Korean traditional diet with good social interactions to prevent chronic diseases.

References

KOSIS (Korean Statistical Information Service) (2017) Vital Statistics in 2016.

KOSIS (Korean Statistical Information Service) (2017) 2016 Population and Housing Census, 2~22.

Lee MS (1992) Modulation of Mutagen Formation by Addition of Spices in Cooking Process of Korean Tastes Meat Food *"Bulgogi"*. *Environmental Mutagens and Carcinogens* 12(2):133–146, 1992

Lee MS (2001) Nutritional Problems of Korean Elderly. *Journal of Korean Medical Association* 44(8):823–842

Lee MS (2002) Dietary Habits and Nutritional Status in Korean Centenarians, In: Park SC, *Korean Centenarians*, Seoul National University Press

Ministry of Health and Welfare · Korea Centers for Disease & Prevention (2017) Korea Health Statistics 2017: Korea National Health and Nutrition Examination Survey (KNHANES VII-2), https://knhanes. cdc.go.kr/knhanes/sub04/sub04_03.do?classType=7, 2019. 10.14

Oh SI and Lee MS (2003) Screening for Antioxidative and Antimutagenic Capacities in 7 Common Vegetables Taken by Korean. *Journal of the Korean Society of Food Science and Nutrition* 32(8):1344–1350

Park SC (2009) *The Story of Centenarians*, SAMTOH Co.

Park SC, Lee MS, Lee JJ and Han GH (2005) *Longevity in Korea: Individuality and Socio-Ecologic Variables in Honam Longlive Area*, Seoul National University Press

Park SO, Park SC, Lee JJ, Han GH, Lee MS, Kwak CS, Song KU and Jeong EJ (2007) *Long-lived Persons and Areas of Longevity in Korea: Changes and Responses*, Seoul National University Press

Seoul National University's Institute of Physical Science and Aging · The Chosun Ilbo (2003) *The Secret of Longevity*, Chosun Ilbo

WHO (2018) 10 facts on ageing and health 2017 update, http://www.who. int/features/factfiles/ageing/en/, 2019. 10.14

3

KOREANS SELECT FOOD ALIGNED AND SUITABLE FOR THEIR CONSTITUTION

CHERL-HO LEE

*Emeritus Professor, Korea
University, Seoul, Korea*

Contents

3.1 Introduction: Origin of Constitutional Diet

Everyone has an approximate knowledge of foods that do not align and fit their bodies. Such an idea may be expressed as a favorite food or disliked food, but there are foods that make people feel upset and even feeling weak when eaten. In other words, there are foods that the body does not accept. Some people are more comfortable with glutinous rice than non-glutinous rice, and in the West, some people have difficulty in digesting it when they eat flour due to bad health effects such as Celiac disease. There are also individuals who cannot eat certain vegetables (for example radish sprouts), people who cannot digest roots after eating root vegetables, and people who avoid meat or certain meats that are different. Attempts to systematically categorize and define these individual differences originated on the Korean peninsula in the late 19th century.

DOI: 10.1201/9781003275732-4

In the 31st year of King Gojong (1894), a medical practitioner in Hamgyung Province, Lee Jema, developed a unique theory of *Sasang* Constitution Typology, not found elsewhere in East Asia. He classified physical types of human beings into four groups: *Taeyang*, *Soyang*, *Taeeum*, and *Soeum*, according to the constitution of individuals, and applied different treatments and diet therapies according to the body constitution. Sasang constitution theory has been accepted as a common sense of health that many Koreans naturally empathize and align naturally with, and therefore influences the individual's food choices in Korea. According to a survey conducted several years ago by Korea University, 90% of the respondents (839 males and females, 20–60 years old) knew Sasang typology, and 88.4% believed that they should eat foods suitable to the individual body type for the prevention and treatment of diseases. About 45.5% of the respondents said they knew their constitution, not only by personal judgment but also evaluated by Chinese doctors (23%) or based on questionnaires (12%) (Lee 2007). Another survey (859 males and females, 20–60 years old) showed that people considered food habits (39.8%) the most important factor for the maintenance of health, followed by exercise (38.8%) and bone physical constitution (13.2%) among other factors like medicine, periodic preventive health checkup, and management of stress (Lee et al. 1996).

In Western countries, the humorism (sanguine, phlegmatic, melancholy, and choleric) of Hippocrates (BC 460–377) and the four humors (black bile, yellow bile, blood and phlegm) of Galen (AD 131–201) have long been used as important diagnostic criteria for medical treatment, but in modern medicine all these concepts are obsolete. In the Far East, there are five phases in the theory of classification and the 25 subtypes are based on Chinese medicine but are rarely applied in diagnosis and dietary therapy. Ayurveda medicine in India divides the constitution into three types (*vata*, *pitta*, *kapha*), which differs from Sasang constitution in that constitution changes according to environments and circumstances.

Korea's Sasang constitution theory is an original cure-based theory that provides specific guidelines for the treatment of diseases and food choices. It is a unique Korean health-targeted medical theory that cannot be found in Chinese medicine or other traditional medicine. This theory has been applied to develop various diets by many people in modern times, and more detailed classification systems are proposed. This chapter also provides an overview of Daoist curing, which is the basis of Korean concept of regimen, *Yin/Yang* and Five Phases Theory of Chinese medicine, and Korean Sasang constitution typology. In addition, this chapter will examine the possibility of connecting Sasang typology with nutrigenomics, which has been recently studied in modern medicine and genomics.

3.2 Daoist Health Concept

In the consciousness of Koreans who share ancient Chinese civilization as descendants of the Eastern Archers Tribe (Dong-Yi), the Daoist Sinseonism (the idea of legendary immortal hermit) originated from the Northeast Asian shamanism and is mixed along with the yin and yang theory of Chinese medicine. Daoism is a native belief that developed around the Shandong peninsula, China, where Dong-Yi lived. The Daoism concepts are divided into Folk Daoism based on old age and Orthodox Daoism established by Chinese philosophers (Lee 2022).

Folk Daoism puts the ultimate goal of life on a disease-free long life and emphasizes harmony of spirit, energy (Ki), and deity, and to become immortal *sinseon* as the highest level. Believing that these goals can be achieved through exercise and training, they emphasize the practices that control breathing, libido, and food. Daoism's ultimate goal is to live a long life in the present world, so regimen and medicine become important training components towards longevity. In terms of Daoist expressions, they can be classified into five categories: *byekgok* (eating uncooked cereals), *bokyi* (medicine method), *josik* (deep breathing), *doin* (massage), and *bangjung* (preserving energy).

In Daoism, the human spirit is seen as being bound to the body. Therefore, the body is sustained by food materials. To enjoy a long life, they recommend reducing the amount and number of meals and avoiding cooked foods. That is how *byekgok* is defined. It is not to eat anything, but to fast and avoid grain. *Bokyi* is a medicine-based method to be fresh or to live for a long time. The drug used as a medicine contains ores such as sulfur and cinnabar, or herbs such as rehmannia (*Rehmannia glutinosa*) and Reishi mushroom (*Ganoderma lucidum*). According to their efficacy, medicines are classified into three groups: upper medicines give a prolonged life to become a heavenly god *sinseon*, middle medicines enhance stamina, and lower medicines cure diseases and expel ghosts. The upper-most medicine is called *dan* or *keumdan*. There are many kinds of *dans*, which are detailed in Taoists' classics, for example, "Pobakja" of Galhong in the early 4th century.

We often say that a strong person is full of vitality. Daoist claims that the source of human vitality is the "Ki" in the body. Emphasis is that "Ki" should be preserved because without "Ki" man will die. *Josik*, which is a general term of *taesik, paegi, tonab,* and *hangki*, is a form of deep breathing. *Doin* is the same method referring to "massage" that was conceived to preserve "Ki" in the body like *josik*. In the book *Ungeup chilchom*, which was compiled by Janggun Bang of the Song Dynasty, there are many methods of *doin*. *Doin* is a method of longevity that many people at that time used to promote health.

Bangjungsul was originally thought to be one of the ways of preserving the body's energy, such as *doin* and *josik*. For example, "Pobakja" says, "However, even if you take a medicine, you cannot live long without knowing the essence of the *bangjung*. Those who want to have immortality should work hard to obtain this method" (vol. 8). Harmonious preservation of the two Ki, yin and yang, in the body is the principle of *bangjungsul*. Various contraindications to *bangjungsul* are also important elements of mental life. Taoist training is a way to maintain health and enjoy longevity, so it can be called the caring method (Lee 2022).

3.3 Principles of an Asian Medicinal Diet

Chinese medicine is based on yin/yang and the five phases theory that have been the root of East Asian culture since ancient times. The yin/yang theory is a theory that observes and deduces nature, including humans, on the principles of yin and yang's relativity, balance, complementarity, and mutual linkage. Yin/yang is the reciprocity of things, such as darkness/brightness, female/male, inside/outside, center/around, weak/strong, empty/full, cold/hot, up/down, plant/animals, death/life, moisture/dry, large/small, coarse/dense, and electron/quantum. The yin/yang relationship is a relative concept of mutual suppression and rebuttal, interdependence, mutual supplement for equilibrium, and inter-conversion, and there is no absolute yin and yang.

The five phases theory divides the nature of things into wood, fire, earth, metal, and water, and generalizes their interrelationships. It is describing or predicting the way of interaction. This is a different concept from the fundamental elements of things (earth, air, fire, water) in ancient Greek science, suggesting a way of interaction, not matter itself as it is in Greek philosophy (Magner 1992). The five-way interaction method is to establish the relationship and process between generation and suppression, as shown in Figure 3.1. The relationship of generation is that water causes trees to grow, wood burns fire, fire makes ashes or earth, and earth is the source of metal, and when metal is heated it flows like water. The relationship of the suppression is that water extinguishes fire, fire dissolves metal, a metal axe cuts wood, a wood plow grinds earth, and dams made of earth stop the flow of water.

Table 3.1 shows the taxonomy of components by five phases. According to this classification, the sour taste, liver, bile, and eyes belong to the same wood, and in the generation of relationships, sour taste helps the heart function, but suppresses the function of the spleen. Bitter taste belongs to the fire, such as the heart, small intestine, tongue, and protects the spleen and inhibits the function of the lungs. This relationship setting is common sense, but it is not yet scientifically interpreted or proved.

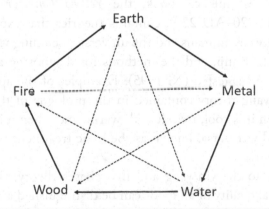

Figure 3.1 The relationship of generation (-) and suppression (- -) in the five phase theory (Lee 2004).

Table 3.1 Classification of the qualities of matter according to the five phases theory

Phases	Taste	Color	Weather	Season	Direction
Wood	Sour	Bright blue	Windy	Spring	East
Fire	Bitter	Deep red	Hot	Summer	South
Earth	Sweet	Yellow	Humid	Late summer	Middle
Metal	Spicy	White	Dry	Fall	West
Water	Salty	Black	Cold	Winter	North

Phases	Organ	Digestion	Sensory Organs	Body	Emotions
Wood	Liver	Bile	Eyes	Tendons	Anger
Fire	Heart	Small intestine	Tongue	Blood vessels	Joy
Earth	Spleen	Stomach	Mouth	Flesh	Love
Metal	Lung	Large intestine	Nose	Hide/Skin	Sadness
Water	Kidney	Bladder	Ears	Bones	Fear

Yin/yang and the five phases theory are the harmony of the two opposite properties of negative and positive of things, and creation, operation, and movement of the universe in terms of five phases: wood, fire, soil, metal, and water. It is the philosophical background of Chinese medicine that originated from the Chinese theoretical system that explains the mutual relationship of generation and suppression of the things. Its origin is derived from the inscription on bones and tortoise carapaces, and it is argued that it goes back to the founder of divinity, Bokyi, by the *Book of Changes* (BC 3000). It is a theoretical system that has been used for divinity and medicine in ancient China.

China's oldest medical book, the *Yellow Emperor's Classics of Medicine* (BC 220–AD 220), contains theories that explain the relationship between humans and the universe, including yin/yang, five phases, and 12 Kanji, and the methods for diagnosing and treating the disease are suggested (Ni 1995). Examples of the application of the yin and yang theory contained in the prologue of the *Emperor's Book* are when it is cool, treat it with warm, and when it is cold, treat with hot, and vice versa, known as the basic treatment of cool, cold, warm, and hot.

According to the yin/yang and five phases theory, the nutrition and functional quality of all foods can be distinguished and judged by their properties and tastes. The nature of food is divided into cold (yin or Eum), neutral or warm (yang). Eum properties also represent the substance of matter such as nutrients, while yang represents energy and functions such as calories. The taste of food is divided into five flavors of the five phases (sour, bitter, sweet, pungent, and salty). Flavors are linked with internal organs toward the generation and suppression relationship. The basic idea of nutrition and diet therapy is to think that eating a balanced combination of food's yin and yang properties and five tastes is good for maintaining health and a balanced diet. Inclining to one property or taste is not healthy.

In the "Shin Nong's Materia Medica," which has come down as a classic of Chinese pharmacology, there are three kinds of drugs.

Upper medicines: 120 kinds of non-toxic foods that can be consumed for a long time like food.

Middle medicines: Toxic but low in level, about 120 species for chronic diseases.

Lower medicines: About 125 species for acute illnesses due to their high toxicity.

This is a good representation of the concept of "food and medicine which have same origin" in oriental medicine that food is the best medicine. This toxicological and pharmacological knowledge is valuable clinical data from thousands of years of living experience.

The *Yellow Emperor's Classic of Medicine* was first introduced to the Korean peninsula in the third year of King Pyungwon of Goguryeo (AD 561). Since then, literature on Chinese medicine was introduced to Korea during the Three Nations period and Koryo Dynasty. At the level of Korean traditional medicine with shamanism and Daoist background, Chinese medicine comparatively would have been a very high scientific method and had a great influence on people's knowledge of natural science and medical treatment regimen skills.

3.4 Development of Eastern Medicine (*Donguihak*) and Sasang Typology

Ancient medicine on the Korean peninsula seems to have been closely influenced by Chinese ancient medicine through frequent exchanges with China since the late Gojoseon (ca. BC 200). The Yellow Emperor's Classic of Medicine describes that stone acupuncture was introduced from the East. It can be observed that traditional medicine was developed since Gojoseon periods with discoveries of stone acupuncture and bone acupuncture that were used in the past. In addition, a lot of good medicines were produced in ancient Korea, and the effects of Korean drugs were listed in Chinese herbal medicine books, and treatment prescriptions using these drugs were also recorded. In addition, the Japanese "Uisimbang" document cited the Korean medicine prescriptions such as "Silla-Bubsabang" and "Baekje-Sinjipbang." It was clearly recorded and inferred that the ancient medicine of Korea spread to China as well as Japan.

The ancient medicine of Korea has been developed mainly as a medicinal practice concept through private experiences. In the Three Kingdoms era, there were prescriptions such as Goguryeo-Nosabang, Baekje-Sinjipbang, and Silla-Bubsabang. There were several books such as Jejung-ibhyobang, Hyangyak-gugeupbang, and Dongingyunghombang in the Goryeo Dynasty.

In the Joseon Kingdom, by the name of King Sejong, Roh Jungrye and Park Yundeok collected all domestic medicine and civilian experiences passed through the Three Kingdoms and Goryeo Dynasty. Over the years, the king had compiled 85 volumes of Hyangyak-jipseongbang. It contains 10,706 experienced prescriptions and 1,476 methods of acupuncture and moxibustion, which were widely used in royal courts and civilians at that time. King Sejong was not satisfied with the "Hyangyak-jipsangbang" and ordered 16 people, including Yu Sung-won and Jeon Soonui, to gather all medical knowledge of the time and lay the groundwork for medical therapy development in Korea. With 153 kinds of dictates and even Buddhist rituals from India, 266 books were completed in Euibang-ryuchwi in three years.

Euibang-ryuchyi is a collection of all theories and pharmacies of medicines used at that time, classified into generalizations and symptom classification, and inventions re-configured, refined, and edited by Korea's own system. This book is a huge document with 80 categories and a total of about 10,000 items, and a valuable material to view and observe the whole picture of Eastern medicine. With the compilation of Hyangyak-jipsungbang and Euibang-ryuchwi, the basis of Eastern medicine research, including all domestic and Chinese medical theories, was integrated and advanced.

In 1596 (29th year of Seonjo, Chosun Kingdom), under the name of Seonjo, Yang Yesoo and Heo Jun established a compilation office in the royal hospital, and published a masterpiece of medicine book, *Dongui-bogam* (AD 610). As the basis of agreement, Heo Jun emphasized that the basis of medicine is in spirit, ki, and deity, and he put the relations on this basis to align the physiological functions and disease symptoms of various organs in internal medicine (*Naegyung*) section, which was not shown in other medicine books at that time. In other words, the medicine's prime purpose is to find a health and cultivation of spiritualty, and drug use is the next layer of solution. In particular, he emphasized the importance of regimen in the Naegyung section, and emphasized the importance of dietary regimen supplementing the four elements that make up the body: spirit, ki, deity, and blood.

In addition, in the introduction of Naegyung section he said, "Dao is based on clean mind and discipline, while medical practice uses drug and acupuncture. Tao has gained its spirit, and medicine integrating overall care." Heo Jun's *Dongui-bogam* is highly regarded as an original Eastern medical book developed by adding traditional folk medicine to Chinese medicine. Under the well-organized structure, *Dongui-bogam* rejected the absurd and fanciful medical theory that was common in oriental medicine and pursued the ultimate reason in medicine that aimed and grasped to gather all kinds of knowledge of the medical field at that time. It is a compilation of the spirit of Dao respecting overall welfare and practicality. Therefore, this book not only focused the pathway of Asian medicine until the 17th century but also became the source of Eastern medicine, which is highly regarded worldwide and established the original medical theory of Korea.

Eastern medicine developed further during the 18th and 19th centuries and was developed by Lee Jema into a unique ideology of medicine not found elsewhere in East Asia. *Dongui-susebowon* is a compilation of Sasang (four constitutions) medical theories written by Lee Jema, a medical practitioner of Hamheung in 1894. Lee Jema classified human constitution into four types according to the physical and mental properties, *Taeyang, Soyang, Taeeum,* and *Soeum,* and suggested the use of different treatments according to the patient's constitution even with the same disease. He also emphasized

Sasang diet therapy by the constitution theory. Sasang constitution typology is a groundbreaking theory out of the traditional oriental medicine that focuses on the constitution of the sick without relying on the conventional theory of yin/yang and five phases theories. It was mainly based on the northern province Hamgyeong-do region in Korea.

The book *Susebowon* was made in four volumes in two books printed as wood blocks, currently in the library of Korea University. The contents are divided into seven chapters: Seongmyungron, Sadangron, Hwakchungron, Jangburon, Uiwonron, Gwangjeseol, and Sasangin-byeonjeungron. In Sasangron, people of the four constitutions are classified and explained in relation to the characteristics of organs as follows:

Men of Taeeum: Large liver and small lung (strong liver function, and weak lung and heart function).

Men of Soeum: Large kidney and small spleen (strong kidney function and weak spleen function).

Men of Taeyang: Large lung and small liver (strong lung function and weak liver function).

Men of Soyang: Large spleen and small kidney (strong spleen function and weak kidney function).

Sasang medicine is a representative theory that characterizes Eastern medicine and has since been studied and applied by many people. The most difficult aspect of Sasang typology is that it is not easy to determine the classification of an individual's constitution accurately and reproducibly. Lee Jema mainly relied on feeling the pulse (pulse diagnosis), but it was not properly transmitted to the later generations. The classification of constitution can be made according to the physique, personality, and taste of a person. The biopsychological characteristics of a Taeyang man are muscular and progressive and creative. A Taeeum man, on the other hand, is large, feminine, quiet, and conservative. A Soyang man is small, active, and outgoing, while a Soeum man is small, quiet, and introverted (Chae et al. 2003).

3.5 Classification of Sasang Constitution Types

Diagnosis for Sasang constitution types include methods using a diagnostic device and a method of discrimination through a questionnaire. As a method using a diagnostic device, a method of detecting and analyzing pulse waves, a method of analyzing morphological features of a face, a method of discriminating fingerprints, and a method of analyzing video and audio signals have been reported, but no method gives reliable and satisfactory results.

A questionnaire method containing 105 questions (QSCC) was developed by Kyung Hee University, College of Korean Medicine in 1993, and QSCC (II) consisting of 121 questions in 1995, and the QSCC (II)+ consisting of 54 questions in 2001. However, the number of questions were too high, and the reproducibility or reliability was not satisfactory (Chae et al. 2003). In 2006, a method containing 50 questions (TS-QSCD) was developed by dividing yin and yang constitutions first and then classifying the four constitutions.

Recently, the Korea Institute of Oriental Medicine has developed a 15-item short-term Sasang Constitution Diagnosis Questionnaire (KS-15) based on body type, personality, and micro symptoms (Baek et al. 2015), and has increased the utilization by creating a web-based constitution diagnosis system (Park et al. 2017). However, these questionnaires also have a problem that the test confidence does not exceed 70%. The Institute of Oriental Medicine has recently developed and used an integrated constitution diagnosis system (SCAT) to conduct objective and comprehensive constitution diagnosis by inputting facial photos, voice recording files, body shape information, and questionnaire on the web (So et al. 2016).

Confidence of Sasang constitution diagnosis devices and analytical methods is mainly based on the judgment of Sasang constitution experts, but the agreement and validity of diagnosis among experts confirming the investigations are at 60% (Baek et al. 2014). Therefore, there is an urgent need for the development of biochemical markers that can objectively discriminate the four constitutions to overcome differences in observational judgement of constitution experts.

Recently, studies to classify constitutions using marker genes have been attempted. Korean medical students were tested for their association with genes involved in antioxidant activity, immune response,

ATP synthesis, and protein degradation by collecting blood from students who received the same constitution in Asian medicine's clinic and questionnaire (QSCC II). Genes p450 2D6, 2C9, IA2, and SOD2 have been reported to be associated with Sasang constitution (Park 2004). In particular, it was confirmed that the SNP distribution pattern varies depending on the constitution. Of course, these findings are just the beginning, but more research is needed to classify people into four constitutions by genetic analysis (Lee 2007).

3.6 Constitutional Food Based on Sasang Medicine

Although the classification of the constitution is inaccurate and low in reproducibility, many studies on food classification by Sasang constitution have been conducted, and many people are eating foods that are suitable for their constitution. Table 3.2 is an example of the list of foods suitable for each constitution suggested by a research team at Kyung Hee University, College of Korean Medicine (Kim et al. 1995). The reliability of this classification is not scientifically confirmed, but it shows the characteristic concept of food regimen of Koreans derived from the tradition of Sasang medicine.

In addition, there are a variety of data on constitution-based foods. For example, Dr. Lee Myung-bok, an honorary professor at the Seoul National University School of Medicine, developed the O-ring test, classifying an individual's body constitution and accordingly created a list of foods that are suitable or not suitable for each constitution (Lee 1989).

Heo (2005) divides the constitution into yin and yang and suggested a diet for patients according to his unique theory of the yin and yang classification and food application. He suggests that yang people should eat yin foods and yin people vice versa. The constitution of individuals is evaluated by a questionnaire about psychological, physiological, and morphological characteristics, in addition to the O-ring test. An example of foods suitable for the people of different constitutions is as follows.

Foods suitable for a yang constitution: green beans, wheat, barley, legumes, cabbage, lettuce, sweet potatoes, eggplant, spinach, pumpkin, burdock, perilla leaves, cucumber, duck, seaweed, banana, persimmon, jujube, pear, tangerine, grape, strawberry, melon, tuna, pork, dog meat,

Table 3.2 An example of Sasang food list (Kim et al. 1995)

	TAEYANG	SOYANG	TAEEUM	SOEUM
Cereals	Buckwheat	Barley, red beans, mung beans, barnyard millet, sesame	Soybeans, Job's tears, sugar, wheat, wheat flour, great millet, perilla, sweet potato, common millet, peanut	Glutinous rice, hulled millet, glutinous millet, potato
Fruit	Kiwifruit, grapes, persimmon, cherries, Chinese quince	Watermelon, Korean melon, strawberries, banana, pineapple	Chestnuts, pear, walnuts, gingko nuts, pine nuts, apricot, plum	Apple, mandarin, orange, peach, jujube
Vegetables	Water shield, pine needles	Cucumber, Chinese cabbage pumpkin, lettuce, eggplant, sow thistle, edible burdock bamboo shoot, Asian plantain	Radish, bellflower root, Indian lotus, taro, hemp, bracken, lanceolate root, shiitake mushroom, ear mushroom, matsutake mushroom, Umbilicaria esculenta (rock tripe)	Water dropwort, Welsh onion, garlic, black pepper, ginger, spinach, carrot, red pepper, crown daisy, onion, mustard
Seafood	Oysters, abalone, conch, shrimp, crucian carp, crab, sea slug, mussels	Flatfish, puffer, turtle, crawfish, carp, snapping turtle, snakehead fish	Freshwater snail, codfish, yellow corvina, small octopus, brown croaker, herring, squid, brown seaweed, laver, kelp	Alaska Pollack, loach, eel, snake, catfish
Meat products		Pork, eggs, duck	Beef, milk	Chicken, lamb, dog meat, pheasant, goat, sparrow meat

sea fish, salted fish, soybean oil, perilla oil, rapeseed oil, green tea, black tea, beer, and wine.

Foods suitable for a yin constitution: rice, glutinous rice, sorghum, millet, corn, radish, potatoes, carrots, onions, leek, tomatoes, pineapples, peaches, watermelons, apples, plums, chestnuts, pine nuts, walnut, sesame oil, corn oil, garlic, pepper, ginger, curry, beef, milk, chicken, duck, lamb, egg, freshwater fish, *Ganoderma lucidum*, ginseng, deer antler, corn tea, ginger tea, rice wine, and *Makgeolli* (Korean turbid rice beer).

Heo Bongsu's food classification is like that of the Kyung Hee University Korean Medicine (Table 3.2). He opened a comprehensive medical center and hired doctors to diagnose patients' diseases and to cure them with diet. There is also a restaurant that provides food for each constitution.

In the 1980s, Kwon Dowon, a medical doctor in Seoul, used eight constitution medicines (*Mokyang, Mokeum, Toyang, Toeum, Geumyang, Geumeum, Suyang,* and *Sueum* constitution). Baek (2000) divided people into 28 constitutions starting from Sasang typology and recommended diets suitable for each constitution. This tendency to further subdivide the constitution is because the classification of the four constitutions is not accurate and the reproducibility is low. For this reason, few people in the scientific community, including the food scientists in Korea, study a diet based on Sasang typology.

3.7 Sasang Typology and Nutrigenomics

Recent advances in molecular biology have led researchers to recognize that individual genetic differences can alter the response to ingredients ingested (Milner 2004). It is common to see one person obese and the other normal, even among siblings in a family consuming the same food. These phenomena were attributed to the differences in individual gene composition and drew attention of the scientists to begin to study the relationship between nutrition and genes (Ordovas and Mooser 2004; Kaput 2004). SNPs found in the human genome are estimated to be 3×10^6 and less than 0.1% of the total number of genes (3.2×10^9 bp), but they cause different responses to various diseases and foods eaten. This field of study is called nutrigenetics. The concept of nutritional genetics has many close parallels conceptually to Sasang medicine (Lee 2007).

Ingested food can also affect the genetic traits of the human body, causing induced epigenetic changes, and this field of study is called nutrigenomics. Eventually, the nutrients we eat cause changes in our genotype on an·ongoing basis, resulting in changes in the associated protein activity (proteomic effects), metabolite changes (metabolomic effects), and changes in diseases and health conditions (phenotype). Epigenetic changes may occur depending on the nutritional component ingested and, consequently, hyperlipidemia, obesity, and diabetes may occur. One can also prevent or treat these diseases by avoiding or eating certain nutrients. In particular, many studies have been conducted on the relationship between heart disease and food intake (such as response to fat and sugar). However, the exact mechanism of specific nutritional and epigenetic variations is not yet known. This is because the complexity of the genome changes and the function of many genes is not fully investigated yet. Furthermore, symptoms and human responses are affected by so many variables. Moreover, the method of applying the individual differences according to the constitution as a variable is not yet established.

As mentioned previously, if genetic analysis enables reproducible constitution-based classification, it can open a significant, exciting opportunity of a constitution-specific (Sasang) food list accumulated through human experiential experiments of thousands of years (Lee 2007). This is expected to greatly reduce the experimental error on the functional food research and to reduce the cost of building and validating scientific proof. Sasang medicine is indispensable for the development of customized foods for today's 100-years longevity-based healthy life and will be a powerful and exciting practical approach that can allow Korean food-based longevity concepts to lead the world in this field.

References

Baek SH (2000) *Healing diseases with food suitable for individual's constitution.* Seoul: Taeung Publisher.
Baek YH, Jang ES and Lee SW (2014) Evaluation on the consistency and validity of the classification of constitution by Sasang medicine experts. *Journal Constitutional Medicine* 26:295–303.

Baek YH, Jang ES Lee SW, Park GH, Ryu JY and Chin HJ (2015) Development and validity of a simplified Sasang constitution questionnaire (KS-15) based on the physical, personality and diseases characteristics of individuals. *Journal Constitutional Medicine* 27:211–221.

Chae H, Lyoo IK, Lee SJ, Cho S, Bae H, Hong M and Shin M (2003) An alternative way to individualized medicine: psychological and physical traits of Sasang Typology. *Journal Alternative and Complementary Medicine* 9(4):519–528.

Heo BS (2000) *Food horoscopes suitable for my body.* Seoul: KBS Film Producer.

Heo BS (2005) *Healing diseases with diet.* Seoul: Garim Publisher.

Kaput J (2004) Diet-disease gene interactions. *Nutrition* 20:26–31.

Kim JY, Kim CW, Koh BH and Song IB (1995) Justification and usage of food classification according to body constitution. *Journal Constitutional Medicine* 7:263–279.

Lee MB (1989) *Natural foods, body constitution and food.* Korea: Medical Insurance Corp.

Lee CH (2004) Functional food of interest to ASEAN: from traditional experience to modern production and trading. *Food Science Biotechnology* 13(3):390–395.

Lee CH (2005) Functional food from traditional experience to modern production, Fi Asia-China Conference, 1–2 March 2005, Shanghai, China.

Lee CH (2007) Harmonization of Eastern and Western health knowledge: Nutrigenetics and Sasang Typology. *Food Science Technology Research* 13(2):85–95.

Lee CH (2018) *History of Korean food.* Seoul: Jayu Academy.

Lee CH (2022) *Korean food and foodways, the root of health functional food.* Springer Nature, Singapore.

Lee CH and Lee CY (2003) *Paradigm shift: Harmonization of Eastern and Western food systems, in bioprocesses and biotechnology for functional foods and nutraceuticals.* pp. 415–425. New York: Marcel Dekker.

Lee EJ, Ro SO and Lee CH (1996) A survey on the consumer attitude toward health food in Korea (I) Consumer perception on health and food habit. *Korean Journal Dietary Culture* 11(4):475–485.

Magner LN (1992) *A history of medicine.* New York: Marcel Dekker.

Milner JA (2004) Molecular targets for bioactive food components. *Journal of Nutrition* 9:134.

Ni M (1995) *The yellow emperor's classic of medicine.* Boston: Shambhala Publisher.

Ordovas JM and Mooser V (2004) Nutrigenomics and nutrigenetics. *Current Opinion in Lipidology* 15:101–108.

Park DI, Jin HJ and Park KH (2017) Korea Sasang constitutional diagnostic questionnaire (KS-15) based on internet web to improve validity of questionnaire. *Journal Constitutional Medicine* 29:224–231.

Park SS (2004) *Fundamentals of genomics. In Founding Symposium of the Korean society of Clinical Genomic Medicine.* Korea: Korea University, Seoul. 5 December 2004.

So, JH, Kim, JE, Nam, JH, Lee, BJ, Kim, YS, Kim, JY and Do, JH (2016) Sasang Constitution Analysis Tool (SCAT). *Journal Constitutional Medicine* 28:1–10

4

THE ANSWER FOR A HEALTHY LIFE IS A KOREAN TRADITIONAL DIET

DAE YOUNG KWON

Hoseo University, Korea Academy of
Science and Technology

Contents

DOI: 10.1201/9781003275732-5

4.1 Introduction

Many people are interested in ethnic foods because of the ease of global travel and interest in the wider world culture. As a result, Korean diets are emerging as a favorite and important cuisine of interest around the world due to its long history and healthiness. Many ask, what is the nature of Korean diet in addition to history, culture, and health (Kwon et al. 2017a)? In the chapter on "Korean Diet and Their Tastes" in the book of *Korean Functional Foods* (Kwon and Chung 2018) or "Diet in Korea" in the book of *Handbook of Eating and Drinking* (Kwon 2020), these concepts were initially discussed. Korea has developed a unique food culture connected to its long agricultural history. In Korea, other lifestyles such as living style in a dwelling or house and style of clothes have totally changed to a Western style; however, eating and diet style are conserved with traditional ways of eating. In modern times, the Korean family still prefers the Korean diet with traditional ways of eating at their homes and even in restaurants, including the younger generation. Only the kitchen for cooking and methods are modernized. Recently, global interest in Korean food, especially its relevance of health benefits, has greatly increased. However, there are insufficient resources and research published on the characteristics and definitions of Korean cuisine. Although the Korean diet (K-diet) has been widely discussed with regards to raw ingredients, traditional cooking methods and technology, fundamental principles, and knowledge, it would be valuable to preserve the traditional methods and knowledge of Korean foods rather than focus on the raw materials themselves. Korean meals have historically been served with *bap* (cooked rice), *kuk* (dishes with broth), kimchi, and *banchan* (side dishes) to be consumed at the same time. As traditionally baking or frying are not common methods, Koreans tend to use fermentation, boiling, blanching, seasoning, and pickling as the key methods of food preparation. Among these methods, the most characteristic method is fermentation. The process of fermentation enriches food flavors and preserves foods.

Korea, located in Northeast Asia, has an agricultural history that has continued for more than 5,000 years, despite its proximity to China. The Han Chinese, who founded the Three Kingdoms and Qin, Tang, Song, and Ming Dynasties, developed their own language and controlled China until the Qing Dynasty emerged. Korea, from Kochosun and, the period of the Three States (including Kokuryo, Baekje, and Silla) to Koryo and Chosun, maintained independence from China and developed a unique culture and language (Woo 2018). Linguistically, the Korean language belongs to the Altaic language group along with the Japonic, Mongolic, Tungusic, Hungarian, and Finnish languages. Moreover, the Mongolian spot, slate grey nevus by congenital dermal melanocyosis on the surface of skin in infants, that is prevalent among Koreans, suggests biological differences between Koreans and Chinese. Likewise, the Korean food culture has also developed distinctly from Chinese cuisine (Chung et al. 2019).

According to Kwon (2015, 2019), the development of food technology was prompted by the desire to preserve food resources and to eat delicious food and meals in addition to eating safely. For example, in China, frying and pickling were the prevalent methods in reducing water content (a_w) to protect against microbial spoilage of food and to increase various tastes. In contrast, the limited production of cooking oils in Korea led to the development of the fermentation process for food preservation, which utilizes effective microorganisms against microbial spoilage. While milk was the main ingredient in fermented products, such as cheese and yogurt, in countries with strong livestock industries as in Western countries, the main ingredients in Korean fermented foods were plant-based such as grains and vegetables. This was due to their settled lifestyle and focus on agriculture. Korean foods have developed from the necessity of eating safely and deliciously while preserving them during hot summers and long, harsh winters on the Korean peninsula, characterized by rocky ocean fronts on the east, south, and west, and by rugged mountains in the north. This geographical isolation from neighboring countries and the distinct weather allowed the early Korean people to develop the most enduring cultural legacies of the Korean diet. In this environment, salted beans, fish, and vegetables were preserved by fermentation. Historically, Koreans have made various *jang* (fermented soy products) (Kwon 2022, Shin and Jeong 2015, Yang et al. 2011), including *kanjang* (soy sauce), *doenjang* (soybean paste), and *kochujang* (red pepper paste), and diverse types of kimchi (Jang et al. 2015) with vegetables. These unique fermentation techniques are examples of authentic Korean food (Kwon et al. 2014). All these fermented *jang* and kimchi are essentials for Korean foods to be tasty, to eat delicious meals, and to swallow and digest it well.

Korea overall has developed unique foods as well as an authentic and original food culture that is fundamentally distinct from Chinese or Japanese food cultures. Food is one of the key elements of culture and presents possibilities for promulgation of various cultural contents. However, this effect has been diminished by a lack of cohesive definitions and concepts in Korean food culture. Therefore, it is necessary to establish consistent definitions and concepts to be used in relation to the Korean diet.

4.2 Definition of Korean Diet (K-diet)

The establishment of consistent definitions and concepts in Korean food (K-food) should be based on systematic and scientific research to promote its health benefits globally. For that, scholars of the food and nutritional sciences have collaborated and announced the "Seoul Declaration on K-diet: Korean Heritage and Healthiness." In the post-industrial age, culture is one of the key elements of a country's competitiveness in the global market. Therefore, this chapter will discuss definitions, characteristics, representative K-foods that have been introduced in the Seoul declaration, and embody fundamental aspects of a Korean meal (Kwon 2016).

The K-diet (Korean diet) and K-food (Korean food) are two separate concepts. The concept of a K-diet is used to represent traditional Korean food culture, cooking methods, and dietary habits and patterns; K-foods are the food constituents of the K-diet. K-food and K-diet are often described as Korean cuisine, Korean diet, or traditional Korean food. A few elements of defining food culture have been put forward, such as frequently consumed foods, raw ingredients or materials, technology or cooking methods, and the fundamental principles found in the country's dietary patterns. These views place a different emphasis on food and diet.

The first aspect introduced, which views K-foods as frequently consumed foods, would allow popular foods among youth, such as *Jajangmyeon* (noodles with *jang*), pizza, or fried chicken, to be considered K-foods. The criteria of the time period for Korean food would be needed but introduces unneeded complexity. The second idea, which has often been cited by the Korean Ministry of Agriculture, suggests that K-food should be made with ingredients (agricultural products) produced only in Korea (Chung 2015). It is limiting to have K-foods which only reference foods traditionally grown in Korea. It is not acceptable, and practicality is limited because so many crops and vegetables are imported around the world now in a globally linked economy. According to this view, kimchi made from imported cabbage would not be considered K-food. The third view proposes the use of traditional cooking technology as the key element of K-food to overcome this issue. Although it is important to preserve traditional Korean cooking methods, this point of view focuses only on the physical and material aspects of methods. As this view overlooks technological advances and, therefore, for example *doenjang* fermented in jars other than *Hang-ari* (Korean earthenware crock) would not qualify as K-food (Kwon and Chung 2018).

Therefore, when discussing K-food and K-diet, one should focus on whether certain dishes are made with traditionally used ingredients regardless of the origin of the produce, follow traditional cooking methods and principles, and lastly, preserve the spirit behind traditional Korean food practices. The definition of traditional Korean food by Chung (Chung 2015; Chung et al. 2016b) reflects these ideas: "Food made with raw materials or ingredients that have been traditionally used in Korea, or with the similar ingredients, use authentic or other similar cooking methods, have historical and cultural characteristics, and have developed and been passed on through people's lives." This meaning contained in Korean food has been interpreted as consistency, patience, consideration, beauty, and appreciation for arts. In the Seoul declaration, the definition of K-diet represents the interpretation as follows:

> *K-diet is composed of bab (cooked-rice) and kuk, and various banchan with one serving called bapsang. Kimchi is always served at every meal. The principal aspects of K-diet include proportionally high consumption of fresh or cooked vegetables (namul), moderate to high consumption of legumes and fish and low consumption of red meat. Banchan is mostly seasoned with various Jang (fermented soy products), medicinal herbs, and sesame or perilla oil.*
>
> *Kwon 2016*

The traditional ingredients of K-food consist of grains and vegetables; however, oceanic regions have used fish and seaweed. Medicinal herbs such as garlic, green onions, and chili have also been used to enhance flavor/taste and add to the health benefits of food. Korean fermentation technology has played an important role in preserving these food resources, including legumes, vegetables, and fish. Historically, grains, including rice and barley, were the main source of carbohydrates. Legumes and fish provided protein. Vegetable oils made from sesame or perilla served as a main source of fat. As metabolic disorders caused by over-nutrition have become a serious problem in developed countries, the Korean diet can be promoted as a healthy alternative. From a sociocultural perspective, the structure of the traditional Korean meal (Kim et al. 2016), which allows people to share various *banchan*

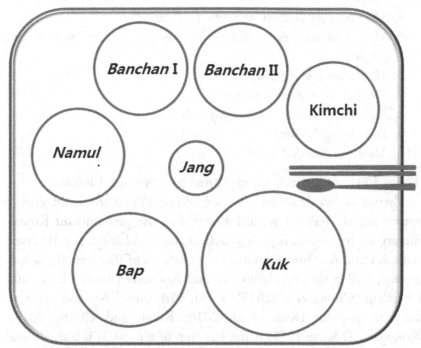

Diagram 1. The Structure of the Traditional Korean Bapsang

Figure 4.1   Diagram of basic *bapsang* in everyday Korean diet. The structure of the traditional Korean *bapsang* (Kwon et al. 2015): *Bap* is served alongside *kuk*, which assists in the swallowing and digestion of the food. In the *bapsang*, *banchan* is comprised of one type of kimchi, one *namul*, one vegetable dish (*Banchan* I), and one high-protein dish (*Banchan* II), usually made from fish or meat as *chim* or *gui*. *Jang*, or salted dishes such as *jangat-ji* and *jeotgal*, are used to season food and stimulate one's appetite. A variety of *bapsang* can be constructed using diverse ingredients and cooking methods depending on the season, regions, andone's preference. Overlapping ingredients and methods allow for well-balanced flavors and nutrients (Kwon 2022; Kwon and Chung 2018).

together, has played an educational role in teaching common etiquette and courtesy to be practiced while eating communal meals (see Figure 4.1 in Kim et al. 2016).

4.3 Characteristics of K-diet

The characteristics of K-diet include:

1. *Various recipes based on rice and grains*
2. *More fermented foods*
3. *More vegetables from wild landscapes and the seas*

4. *More legumes and fish and less red meat*
5. *More medicinal herbs like garlic, green onion, red pepper, and ginger*
6. *More sesame and perilla oil*
7. *Little deep-fat fried cooking*
8. *More meals based on seasonal produce*
9. *Various local cuisines*
10. *More home-cooked meals*

These 10 characteristics are explained in more detail below:

Various recipes based on rice and grains: While the main energy source found in Western cuisine is wheat, the predominant Korean dietary energy source is grains such as rice and barley. *Bap* is served with *kuk* and *banchan* (Figure 4.1). Variations of this format, such as *kukbap*, a dish that combines *kuk* and *bap* served in one bowl, and bibimbap (Chung et al. 2015), a dish with mixed *bap* and *banchan*, are also popular (Kim et al. 2016; Kwon and Chung 2018). *Sungnyung* (Moose 1911) is the last step of a meal. It is a traditional Korean drink made from the roasted crust of rice that forms on the bottom of a pot after cooking rice.

More fermented foods: Throughout the agricultural history of Korea, fermentation technology has been widely used to enrich the flavors of food by utilizing effective microorganisms against microbial spoilage. Fermented soy products, such as *kanjang, doenjang, chong-kukjang* (Kwon 2022; Yang et al. 2011), and *kochujang* are the fundamental ingredients of various sauces and *kuk*. *Doenjang-kuk*, made with vegetables and *doenjang*, is a traditional iconic *kuk*. Kimchi is another representative Korean fermented food known for its authenticity and its health benefit of reducing the activity of harmful bacteria. *Jeotgal* is salted, fermented seafood used to enhance flavor and appetite rather than increase the nutritional value of food (Koo and Kim 2018). As mentioned previously, traditional fermentation technology has been used to intensify flavors in food beyond its role in food preservation.

More vegetables from wild landscapes and the sea: The Korean diet is characterized by high vegetable intake, which is due to the agricultural environment of the country. Vegetables such as lettuce, peppers, carrots, or cucumbers were often consumed raw with sauces made of *kochujang, doenjang, kanjang,* or vinegar, and topped with sesame seeds. Cabbage or spinach were often blanched and seasoned with traditional spices. Both raw and dried vegetables were ingredients for *kuk,* which was flavored with *doenjang* (Kang et al. 2016). Kimchi is the most widely enjoyed vegetable dish in Korea. Korean cuisine also includes various types of seaweed dishes made from laver, green algae, kelp, *Hizikia fusiformis,* and *Capsosiphon fulvescens,* all of which are abundant sources of dietary fiber and vitamins.

More legumes and fish and less red meats: Koreans have enjoyed diverse legumes and nuts such as soybeans, mung beans, red beans, cowpeas, peanuts, walnuts, and ginkgo nuts. Surrounded on three sides by oceans, Koreans have also consumed fish using various techniques to prepare them, such as grilling, boiling in sauce, and marinating. Because lamb, horse meat, beef, and pork were rare in the agricultural environment, the main source of protein intake was poultry, such as chicken and pheasant, but pheasant is rarely used these days.

More medicinal herbs like garlic, green onion, red pepper, and ginger: Compared to the geographically close countries of China and Japan, one of the interesting characteristics of Korean food is the diverse use of *yangnyom* (a kind of seasoning), created with garlic, green onions, red pepper, and ginger (Surh 2003; Na and Surh 2018, Kim et al. 2020). While spices like black peppers have been widely used to hide the unpleasant odors of food in Southeast Asia, medicinal herbs have been used to enhance flavors and increase the food's health benefits (Hur 1610).

More sesame and perilla oils: Historically, the amount of animal-based and vegetable cooking oils produced in Korea was quite limited. While camellia, castor, sesame, and perilla oils were produced in Korea, mainly sesame and perilla oils were used in cooking. With its distinctive aroma, sesame oil was used in *kuk, namul,* and bibimbap. Perilla oil was used in pan-frying foods or making *yukwa* (a puffed rice snack).

Little deep-fat fried cooking: As mentioned previously, deep-frying techniques could not have developed in Korea due to the limited production of animal-based and vegetable cooking oils. Instead, cooking methods such as pan-frying or stir-frying, which did not require large amounts of oil, were developed. *Jeon,* a type of pancake made from flour batter, is the most representative example of this cooking method.

More meals based on seasonal products: Korea has an advanced agricultural industry and four distinctive seasons, which provided abundance and diversity of ingredients. For this reason, its cuisine has developed recipes that use fresh ingredients available in each season. For example, Koreans make fresh kimchi all year round utilizing different varieties of seasonal cabbage, except during the winter, as kimchi is stored underground in jars to control the temperature for fermentation (Jang et al. 2015).

Various local cuisines: Surrounded by oceans on three sides, Korea lacks extensive plains; mountains cover over 70% of its territory. Recipes have been developed based on regional characteristics: grain-based dishes such as bibimbap in the plains (Surh 2003), seafood dishes in oceanic regions (Kim and Jang 2015), vegetable dishes such as *namul* (Lee 2018; Kim et al. 2020) in mountainous regions, and dishes with freshwater fish or clams in regions near rivers. The identification and refinement of these regional recipes and ingredients would be valuable.

More home-cooked meals: The history of agriculture in Korea has shaped a group culture based on family and community. Dedication, communication, and consideration among family members are deeply held values in its culture. As meals are cooked with natural ingredients rather than processed ingredients, usually by mothers, Koreans have believed that food represents a mother's love. This idea has been reflected in the K-diet with *Jipbap* (home-cooked meal) and *umma-sonmat* (the taste of mother's love).

4.4 The Structure of *Bapsang* and Representative K-Diet

4.4.1 The Structure of Bapsang of the K-Diet

As mentioned in previous publications (Kwon et al. 2017a; Kwon and Chung 2018; Kwon 2020), it is crucial to analyze the components of a K-diet and identify representative characteristics of K-foods.

For easy understanding previous publication (Kwon 2016) introduced Korean *bapsang* as follows (Figure 4.1): Korea's traditional meal (*bapsang*) is generally made up of four constituents.

Bap (cooked rice) provides calories, the main source of energy. *Kuk* (soup) allows people to chew and swallow rice, in turn supporting the digestive system. Previously, the word *kuk* was translated into meaning soup; however, *kuk* is quite different from Western soup (Kim et al. 2016; Kang et al. 2016). *Banchan* (side dishes) make up the third element and make the food taste better to support digestion while replenishing the body with nutrition. Usually *namul*, legumes, and fish comprise *banchan*. *Jang* (sauce, *yangnyom*) stimulates people's appetites (Kwon 2022; Shin and Jeong 2015, Hwang et al. 2005). *Yangnyom* includes herbs like garlic, green onions, red pepper, and onions. Unlike spices that are often used to cover or remove unpleasant smells of food, Korean *yangnyom* is used to enhance flavors and increase the health benefits of the foods it is combined with (Kim et al. 2020, Surh 2003, Na and Surh 2018).

The kinds of *bap* (cooked rice) that are used in main dishes include steamed rice, boiled barley, and multigrain rice. As for *kuk*, *doenjang kuk*, *miyok* (sea mustard) *kuk*, and beef *kuk* are commonly eaten. Kimchi is always there as part of *banchan*, as are others, including roasted meat, vegetables, and salad dressed with garlic and chili powder; vegetables served as cooked or fresh *namul*; cooked *namul* seasoned with sesame seed/oil or perilla seed/oil, and fresh vegetables seasoned with vinegar are also served as side dishes. The most basic seasoning used to make the food savory is *kanjang* (fermented soy sauce; *jang* in Korean means fermented soy sauce or paste), *doenjang* (fermented soybean paste), vinegar, *kochujang*, and *jeotkal* (fermented fish sauce from anchovies, shrimp, and other seafood) (Kwon 2022, Shin and Jeong 2015; Koo and Kim 2018). *Jeotkal* can be eaten as a side dish itself and more often is used as seasoning (Hwang et al. 2005; Koo and Kim 2018). In Korea, people drink *sungnyung* (like tea made from leftover scorched rice to surface of pot) to finish off a meal (Moose 1911). By using these four fundamental foods, Korean people have been developing their own unique meals (*bapsang*) by choosing one or more elements in each category even in the food services such as schools and factories.

Key elements of the Korean meal structure have been established and the 100 most representative K-foods have been selected according to these elements (see Table 4.1). Most Korean meals are composed of *banchan* served with *bap*, but they are often misunderstood as main dishes by Westerners. Although some modern

Table 4.1 Categories of elements which construct the Korean diet (Korean *bapsang*) (Fig. 4.1), and representative Korean foods (K-food). Representative K-food will be described in the text briefly (Kwon 2020)

CATEGORY	SUB-CATEGORY	REPRESENTATIVE KOREAN FOODS (K-FOOD)
Bap (main dish)	*Bap*	*Ssalbap* (white rice, brown rice, black rice), *boribap, kongbap, okokbap* (five-grain rice), *nurungji*
	Juk	*Juk* (rice juk), *pumpkin juk, abalone juk, mungbean-juk, red-bean juk*
	One-bowl food	*Bibimbap, theokmandut-kuk (theok-kuk, mandutkuk), kuk-bap, kuksu* (*naengmyeon, kal-kuksu, kong-kuksu, kuksujang-kuk*)
Kuk Tang	*Kuk tang*	*Doenjang-kuk, bukeokuk, kongnamulkuk, miyok-kuk, beat/radish-kuk, torankuk, sundaekuk, fish/maeuntang, Komtang* (*seollungtang, kalbitang*), *haemul-tang, samkye-tang, yukgaejang, choowotang, dakdori* (chicken-dori)-tang
	Chigael Chonkol	*Kimchi-chigae, doenjangchigae, cheongtukjangchigae, sundubuchigae, oiganjeong*
Banchan	*Kimchi*	*Baechukimchi* (*bossamkimchi*), *kkakdugi, oisobagi, chongkak-kimchi, mul-kimchi* (*dongchimi, nabak-kimchi*), *yeolmu-kimchi, gat-kimchi*
	Saengchae	*Saengchae* (radish, cucumber), *juksunkyeojachae, buchu-muchim, dalrae-muchim, miyok-muchim, parae-muchim*
	Sukchae	*Kong* (soybean)-*namul, sikeumchi-namul, doraji-namul, kosari-namul, beoseot-namul, aehobaknamul, gaji-namul, chwi-namul, naengi-namul, gondre-namul, meowideulkkaejeuptang, japchae, tangpyeong-chae* (*muk-muchim*), *gujeolpan*
	Chim	*Kalbichim, suyuk, saengseon-chim, sundae, kaetnip-chim*
	Gui	*Kimgui, saengseon-gui, kalbi, bulgoki, samkyopsal, teok-kalbi, bukeo-gui, deodeok-gui, borigulbi*
	Jorim	*Saengseon-jorim, soegokijang-jorim, kongjaban, yeongeun-jorim, dubu-jorim*
	Jeolim	*Jangat-ji*
	Bokeum	*Myeolchi-bokeum, ojingo-bokeum, jeyuk-bokeum, theokboki, oi-bokeum (oibaetduri)*

	Jeon	Saengseon-jeon, chaeson-jeon (squash, eggplant, burdock, shiitake), hwayangjeok (pasanjeok), pa-jeon, haemul-pajeon, nokdu-bindaeteok, buchu-jeon, dubu-muchim, yuk-jeon
	Hoe	Saengseon-hoe, hongeo-hoe, kang-hoe (green onions, water parsley), dureup-sukhoe
	Dried Banchan	Bukak, ssam (loose leaf lettuce, perilla leaf, crown daisy)
Jang/Yangnyom	**Jang**	Jang (doenjang, chongkukjang, kochujang, kanjang)
	Yangnyom	Yangnyom (green onion, onion, chili, ginger), oil (sesame oil, perilla oil)
	Jeotgal	Jeotgal (shrimp, oyster, pollack roe), Kajamisikhae
Deserts	**Theok, hankwa**	Shaped theok (songpyeon), pounded theok (injeolmi), steamed theok (baekseolki, ssukseolki, siru-theok, jeungpyeon, yaksik), karae-theok, pan-fried theok (hwajeon), boiled theok (gyeongdan), yakkwa
	Drink/Beverages	Sikhye, sujeongkwa, omija-cha, hwachae, sungnyung

Korean restaurants offer food served in courses, the traditional Korean meal is served all at once on the table. One-bowl dishes are not included in the *bap* category in Table 4.1 as one-bowl dishes and rice cake are consumed during busy farming seasons or on special occasions, such as weddings, 60th birthdays, and ancestral rites (Kwon and Chung 2018). Examples of one-bowl meals include *kuksu* (a noodle dish), *kukbap* made from *kuk* and *bap*, bibimbap (Chung et al. 2015) made from *bap* and *banchan* mixed with *jang*, and *theok-kuk* made from *theok* (rice cake) and consumed on New Year's Day. The *kuk* category includes *kuk* and *kuk*-based one-bowl dishes (Kwon and Chung 2018), such as *chigae, jeonkol*, and *tang*. The *banchan* category consists of kimchi, *namul*, and *banchan* made from protein sources such as meat and fish. The *jang* category comprises of *jang*, which is used for seasoning and stimulating one's appetite (Kwon 2020). This includes salted *banchan*, such as *jangat-ji, jeotgal*, and other types of *yangnyom*. Drinks, such as *sungnyung, theok*, and *hankwa* are included in the dessert category. Although this classification is disparate from the traditional Korean meal structure (Yoon 1999), it is helpful for sharing with those who are familiar with the theories and concepts of modern food science. More discourse will be needed to refine this table to effectively bridge this approach between traditional understandings and modern food science.

4.4.2 *The Representative* Bapsang *of K-Diet*

While cuisine from the Korean royal court has been widely studied and is currently served in restaurants, this chapter focuses on food traditionally consumed by the common people. The traditional Korean meal table, or *bapsang*, is categorized by the purpose of the meal. It differs depending on whom the meal is for and the occasion for the meal. For example, a meal for guests would be different compared to a meal for elders of a family. Food consumed during celebrations such as birthdays and weddings would not be the same as food for funerals and ancestral rites. Each Korean holiday, including *Seollal* (New Year's Day), *Boreum* (day of the full moon), *Chusok* (Korean Thanksgiving Day at full-moon in mid-autumn), *Dano* (the fifth day of the fifth month of the year according to the lunar calendar), *Chilseok* (July 7th in the lunar calendar), and *Dongji* (winter solstice), are celebrated with unique and seasonal dishes such as spring *bapsang*, summer *bapsang*, autumn *bapsang*, and winter *bapsang*).

As written previously (Kwon and Chung 2018), the Korean *bapsang* varies according to the purpose of the meal. This section introduces *Jongwol Daeboreumsang* (a kind of *bapsang* at first full moon of the lunar year) as an example of a holiday meal, and *Kawul Bapsang* (*bapsang* for autumn) as an example of a seasonal *bapsang* (a kind of *bapsang* served at autumn).

Jeongwol Daeboreum Bapsang: Koreans traditionally used the lunar calendar, so a full moon was considered to have a special importance and it was believed that days with a full moon were filled with yin/yang (see Chung et al. 2015). The celebration of the first full moon, which falls on the 15th day of the lunar calendar, is the biggest holiday along with the eighth full moon, *Chusok*. During the celebration, people wish for good health and fortune in the upcoming year by playing traditional games and sharing meals (Figure 4.2). In the morning of *Jeongwol Daeboreum*, people make *okokbap* with five grains (glutinous rice, red beans, beans, sorghum, and millet) and dried *namul* (bracken, mushroom, eggplant, squash, cucumber, dried radish greens, and aster), which is preserved from the past year to be consumed in the winter. These dried *namul* are first soaked in water, blanched, then seasoned or stir-fried. Dried *namul* is a great source of nutrients, dietary fiber, minerals, and vitamin D, which is difficult to source during the winter season. Cracking *Bureom* (nuts, such as walnuts and ginkgo nuts) is another popular tradition believed to prevent skin problems through the consumption of unsaturated fatty acid. People also enjoy the custom of *Kwibalkisul*, which is sharing a type of rice wine together while wishing good fortune for the year ahead. *Kwibalki* means "ear-quickening."

Kawul Bapsang: Bapsang served in the fall follows the basic structure of the K-diet described in Figure 4.3. This structure of *bapsang* was established in the Chosun Dynasty. It consisted of *bap* made with new-harvest rice and other grains, *kuk*, kimchi, and various *banchan*. Depending on the available ingredients, mothers would make *banchan* using an appropriate cooking method, such as the ones suggested in Table 4.1, and then they would season with *jang*, garlic, green onions, ginger, red pepper powder, and sesame or perilla oil. *Banchan* typically consists of 80% *namul* dishes and 20% high-protein dishes that are

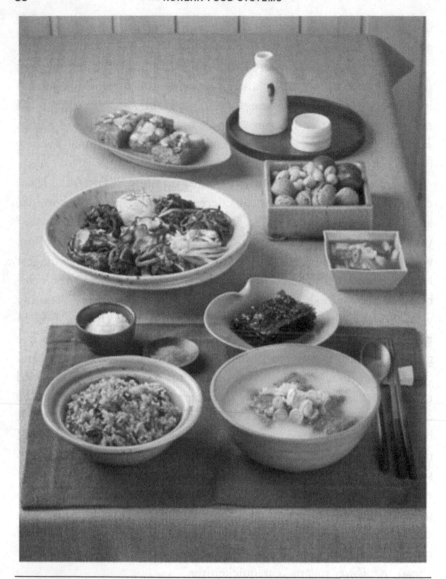

Figure 4.2   *Jeongwol Daeboreum-sang*: This *bapsang* is served on *Jeongwol Daeboreum-sang*, the 15th day of the lunar calendar. It consists of *okokbap, gomkuk,* and *namul* from the past year (eggplant, bracken, squash, dried radish greens, aster, pepper, cucumber, mushroom), *kimgui, na-bakkimchi, yaksik,* and *bureom*. People share *kwibalgisul* with the meal and wish for good health and fortune in the upcoming year. *Kwibalgi* means "ear-quickening" (Kwon and Chung 2018).

made with meat, fish, eggs, or tofu. The varieties of *banchan* offer a healthy, balanced diet that is rich in nutrients and phytochemicals. All dishes are served on a table at once so people can consume them based on their need and preference (Kwon and Chung 2018; Kwon 2020).

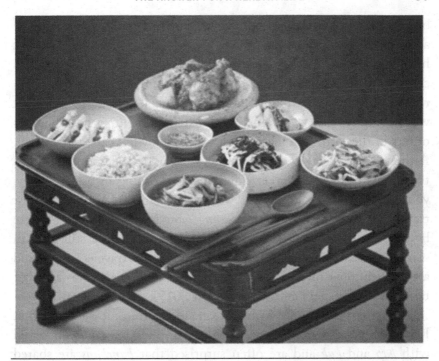

Figure 4.3 *Kawul Bapsang*, an example of a simple seasonal *bapsang*. New-harvest rice, *doenjangkuk, dakdori-tang, dububuchim, beoseot-namul, paraemuchim*, and *chongkakkimchiare* served with *Kanjang*.

4.5 Values of Korean Diet

When it comes to the values embedded in Korean food, which has traditions that date back thousands of years, three essential things come to mind. The first is respect and looking out for others, the second is balance and harmony, and the third is being healthy.

4.5.1 Respect and Consideration

When preparing a meal in Korea, it is common to put elders first and cater to their preferences in terms of food selection. All family members sit around the table (*bapsang*) and eat together. Sometimes, a separate meal is served for elders out of respect. When seated around the *bapsang*, other family members wait for elders to pick up their spoons first before beginning to eat. These dining customs, which are a common part of Korean food culture, were borne out of broader cultural norms of mutual respect and looking out for one another. Korea has a long history as an agrarian society, but this history is not filled with abundance. In fact, as recently as the 20th century, some Koreans were forced to sustain themselves on herb roots and tree bark during the Japanese colonial period. Therefore, it was not always easy to obtain a full meal and providing hospitality to others in the form of a meal was a way of showing care and respect. Although the usual greeting in the West is "good morning," it is traditional in Korea to greet elders in the morning by asking "Have you eaten?" In the old days, it was even customary to look out for travelers who were staying at a *sarang-bang* (guest room) in a house by offering them a meal. These cultural traditions are still alive in some rural restaurants in Cholla Province, where travelers are served a full traditional meal. Preparing a K-diet is an elaborate task that takes a lot of respect and work (Kwon 2019).

Westerners unfamiliar with Korean culture think it is strange that Koreans regularly eat meals consisting of nothing but *banchans* served with *bap* and *kuk* and are often surprised that *banchans* are shared together by chopsticks and spoon. Some were critical of the fact that Koreans dip the spoon again in communal dishes such as *tang* and *chigae*. Of course, from a hygiene perspective, this criticism is not ill-founded. However, this is one of the features of the Korean food culture. The influence of this cultural heritage can be seen in res-taurants. When eating in Western restaurants, Westerners tend to order a single dish for each person, while Koreans will order several dishes to share while chatting. This dining culture led to develop-ment in the range of *banchans* that are served with *bap*, the custom of sharing *banchans* between multiple people, and the cultural practice of looking out for others. Eventually, this sharing culture created broader social norms of caring for and giving way to others. Even today, a group of four customers at a Korean restaurant will typically only be given a single menu, while each member of the group receives a menu in Western restaurants.

4.5.2 *Balance and Harmony*

One main difference between Korean food and Western food is that the question is not "What shall we eat?" but "What shall we eat *bap* with?" Selecting *banchans* to pair with *bap* was of vital importance when Koreans in ancient times decided what to serve for a meal. One of the most important questions to consider was balance and harmony (Kwon 2019). People put effort into achieving balance between nutrition and health, vegetables, and meat, and even the colors of side dishes. Sometimes color is more important for food to be mouthwatering. While foods were divided into categories based on the four *qi* and five elements theory (4氣5味論) in China (Ko et al. 2014), ordinary Korean women would naturally seek balance and harmony when preparing meals even if they had no knowledge of this theory. Careful consideration was the balance and harmony given to health depending on who would be eating the meal.

Because Korean food culture developed from the country's agrarian history, nature is an integral element. Therefore, Korean food differs by season, and Koreans developed cultural traditions of praying to nature during natural disasters such as poor harvests, while thanking nature for bumper crops. Because Korea's agriculture and food culture are rooted in the belief that seasonal foods are the healthiest and most natural foods, Korean food is healthy in both biological and cultural terms. Seasonal foods and foods based on the 24 divisions of the lunar calendar demonstrate the way in which Korean food seeks harmony and balance with nature.

While pursuing harmony and balance, Korean food also guarantees the right to choose. By serving *bap* and a variety of *banchans* as part of the same meal, traditional Korean table settings allow each person to choose what they eat based on their personal preferences. Therefore, Korea developed a different "chopsticks culture" from that of China or Japan. This chopsticks culture is a symbolic part of Korean food culture, in which each person can choose from among a variety of *banchans* presented on one *bapsang*. In the Western culture, once the question of "What shall we eat?" has been answered, there is little room for further choices at the table. All orders as a variety of sauces, a variety of side dishes, and cooking style are placed individually before serving. In contrast, because the question of "What shall we eat it with?" is more important in Korean food culture, where each individual can choose what to eat based on their tastes and preferences even after the meal is served at the table and shared. This tradition led to the customs of offering and sharing side dishes (*banchans*) with one's dining companions and respecting and looking out for other people. In fact, the diversity of Korean food should contribute greatly to the harmony and balance of Korean food.

4.5.3 Being Healthy

As leading healthy lifestyles has become an important global trend (Kwon 2018), renowned healthy diets, such as the Mediterranean (Willett et al. 1995) and Nordic (Adamsson et al. 2012) diets, have been studied and promoted globally. Moreover, studies on the French diet have reported an interesting epidemiological observation called the French Paradox (Ferrieres 2004), referencing that French people have low incidence of cardiovascular disease (CVD) despite high consumption of saturated fats in their diet. It is presumed that the French lifestyle and consumption of red wine (containing resveratrol) lower the incidence of CVD (Simini 2000). Of course, consuming resveratrol-rich red wine is not the only reason, the French do not snack, so their intake of salt and fat is reduced. Moreover, moderate drinking of wine with family or friends is related to lowering CVD risk.

Research has suggested that the health benefits of Korean food are due to the diversity of ingredients and cooking methods used in Korean cuisine (Health Magazine 2006). The average life expectancy in Korea is over 80 years, despite the popularity of high-salt dishes such as *kuk*, *tang*, and kimchi. Excessive salt consumption is a risk factor for CVD (cardiovascular disease). This phenomenon has been referred to as the Korean Paradox (Park and Kwock 2015) and some researchers have claimed that the paradox can be explained by the regular consumption of vegetables and the types of salt used in Korean cuisine. Historically, Koreans have used unrefined, baked, or fermented salts, which may have different health effects compared to refined salt in relation to CVD. Research has shown that consumption of fermented foods like kimchi high in salt is not associated with high blood pressure (Song and Lee 2014). Moreover, high potassium intake assists in discharging salt from the body and, as a result, reduces the risk of CVD (Park and Kwock 2015).

As problems of over-nutrition have become prevalent, the Korean diet (Kwon 2020; Kwon et al. 2017a; Kwon and Chung 2018), characterized by the high consumption of *namul* (seasoned vegetable dishes, Lee 2018; Kim et al. 2020) and fermented foods, can have positive health impacts worldwide. While the health benefits of the Korean diet have been supported by research, more resources are needed to further understand the elements of balanced meals in the Korean diet. Although there are some definitions and characteristics of individual dishes available, there is not a holistic approach to categorizing the data to explain the health benefits of Korean food.

4.6 The Tastes of Korean Foods

While there are several ways to describe the characteristics of food, such as smell, taste, color, and nutrient content and composition, the most frequently used is taste (*mat*; 맛). Taste is the sensory impression of food in the mouth with tongue reacting with taste buds along with smell and is trigeminal nerve stimulation. Taste can be defined in both a narrow physiological way and in a broad general sense (Ryu 2015). According to the physiological definition, taste is the chemical sensation produced when a substance reacts with taste receptor cells in the taste buds, which is then transferred through chemical reaction to the central nervous system by way of gustatory nerves. Research has revealed that there are five basic tastes (味): sweet, sourness, salty, bitter, and umami (brothy with spicy blend in Korea, which was found in the 20th century by Japanese scientists) (Bear et al. 2006; Ryu 2015).

However, in some cases, this physiological approach is inadequate to fully explain the characteristics of tastes found in food. Alternatively, taste in a broader sense includes the sense of pain that stimulates somatosensory nerves such as the spiciness of peppers and astringency of persimmons. Experiential characteristics of tastes such as *siwonhan-mat* (Lee et al. 2013; Kang et al. 2016), *kipeun-mat*, and *eolkeunhan-mat* (taste, a little spicy and hot) (Ryu 2015) are also included in taste in this broader sense. In addition, the sense of temperature, such as cool and hot, plays an important role in enjoying food (Choi 2009).

As we have seen, taste is crucial in assessing the quality of food and initiating preference. Generally, flavor (including taste and smell) and quality of processed foods are determined solely by taste sensed through receptors on the tongue. However, there is a unique taste, beyond the chemical or physiological definition of taste, found in traditional foods of various countries. This unique taste, the third taste, is not experienced through gustatory cells. The diverse sensations of food touching soft tissues in the mouth, swallowing food in the throat, digestion in the stomach, and appreciating the color of foods are examples of the third taste (Li et al. 2002). Therefore, to understand the ethnic food of a country, one is required to understand cultural expressions and the components of food found in that country.

4.6.1 Kan

All nations and ethnicities have their own traditional foods and tastes. In most countries, those tastes remained intact at least up until the advent of the industrialization, and unlike in modern times, were not always sweet. In fact, many of these traditional tastes were viewed as inedible by outsiders, who thought such foods had a strange taste. In particular, traditional Korean fermented foods such as kimchi and *doenjang* were difficult for foreigners to eat. Books written by western missionaries a century ago describe the unique foods and tastes found in Korea (Moose 1911).

In Korea, people traditionally used the expressions "*kan* is *matda*" (the level of saltiness is right) and "*kan* is not *matda*" (the level of saltiness is not right) to describe foods as tasty or not. When Korean women wanted to gauge the taste of a *tang, kuk,* or *namul*, they would check to see how the *kan* was (Kwon 2017a; Song 2009). *Kan* was used as the yardstick for measuring taste. Countries in which sugar was hard to find tended to use salt as a seasoning for food. It is easy to forget that salt, not sugar, is the best-tasting ingredient in the world. In Korea, the eldest to even the youngest recognized that salt is the best-tasting material in the world. In the West, people described a food as "sweet" if they liked the taste, but Koreans believed that food was tasty if it was suitably *kan* (salty), and ill-tasting if it was not. Food was considered to have a poor taste if it contained too little salt, while too much salt made it excessively salty and bitter. *Kan* is a typical representative characteristic of harmony and balance of K-diet. Unlike sugar, which has no upper limit, adjusting *kan* by adding extra salt beyond a certain level makes food taste bitter. Therefore, the Korean expressions for delicious and poor tasting is derived from getting the level of *kan* just right.

Sugar tends to override other tastes, while salt mixes with and brings out other traditional tastes. In traditional Korean cooking, care was taken to avoid adding too much salt to create a balanced and harmonized taste. Recent research shows that Korean food is viewed as having "*siwonhan-mat*" (a refreshing taste) only when it contains the correct level of salt (Kang et al. 2016; Jang et al. 2016). Other research suggests that the right level of saltiness makes food taste great, and when people enjoy their meals with the right tastiness and deliciousness it is believed to make them healthier in general.

In addition to salt, *kanjang* (original meaning of *kanjang* is the *jang* which adjusts *kan*) is another common seasoning found in Korean cuisine. Salt helps to bring out the natural taste of foods, and soy sauce is the best complement for producing a pleasant taste. *Kanjang* is made with fermented soybeans, and has a deep, rich taste on its own with protein hydrolysates such as peptides and amino acids. When Koreans used to make *kanjang* in the past, they would describe it as having "*kemi*" if the taste was satisfactory (Kim 1996). Adjusting the taste of the dish or *banchan* with *kanjang* rather than salt is one way to create a unique traditional Korean taste and flavor.

However, as Korea became an industrialized nation, many people, including chefs, began researching how to replace traditional tastes with newer, tastier ones. Therefore, so many countries, including Korea, now add sugar to food. Sugar reigns supreme when it comes to masking the taste or smell of unfamiliar foods and making them taste sweeter. Sugar led to the abandonment of traditional tastes and facilitated the pursuit of a new "taste hegemony" based around sweetness. While salt and *kanjang* require balance and harmony, adding more sugar to food simply makes it sweeter. Currently, globally people have developed a sweet tooth, but this trend has led to excessive consumption of sugar over the last few decades, resulting in severe health problems from diet-linked chronic diseases such as conditions like obesity, diabetes, and cardiovascular disease, which are now prevalent with excess calories in many countries.

4.6.2 Baro-keumat *(The Right Taste by Mother)*

In the sense of relevance to mother, studying traditional Korean food, or K-diet, entails a thorough understanding of the unique tastes of Korean food. Many Koreans feel nostalgia for the flavors found in traditional foods they used to enjoy. For example, many people have strong memories of the unique taste of *doenjang-kuk* (see the section 7 in this chapter) prepared by their mother growing up, which is said to come with *umma-sonmat* (the taste from mother's hands and love) (see section 3 of this chapter). In fact, there are many expressions related to taste in Korean. However, it is unfortunate that many of these traditional flavors have disappeared in the modern era and been replaced with a simplified, universal sweet taste. So, what kinds of expressions are there for the flavors of Korea?

A substantial number of expressions in the Korean language describe *baro-keumat* (the right taste by mother): the third taste or compounded taste (Kim 2008; Lee et al. 2013; Kwon et al. 2017a; Kwon 2020). Lee et al. (2013) have listed the third tastes of Korean food:

Mat-itneun: delicious

Mat-upneun: unsavory

Siwonhan: fresh, pleasureful, and good digestibility

Kipeun (*kemi*): rich and real; the taste which can be realized by the stomach and spiritual in addition to the tongue

Kalkeumhan: a taste feeling cleanliness

Keoljukhan: a taste feeling thick or juicy

Jeongkalhan: a taste feeling neat or nicely presented

Kosohan: a taste feeling delicate or aromatic

Hyangkeuthan: a taste feeling fragrant or fresh

Tatheuthan: a taste feeling warm or heated and comfortable

Sangkeumhan: a taste feeling fresh or refreshed

Chagaun: a taste feeling cool or cold

Neukkihan: a taste feeling repellently or oily (contrarily to *siwonhan*)

Generally, compounded taste refers to a taste created through combinations of the five basic tastes (saltiness, sourness, sweetness, bitterness, and spiciness or umami). However, *baro-keumat* in Korean food indicates combined tastes acquired from the tongue and other organs in the body. For example, *jeongkalhan-mat* and *kalkeumhan-mat* are compounded tastes using taste buds and vision. *Kosohan-mat*, *hyangkeuthan-mat*, and *sangkeumhan-mat* are tastes using taste buds and smell. The combinations of pain, taste, and temperature are also found in expressions related to Korean food. Of all *baro-keumat* in Korean food, *siwonhan-mat* (Bear et al. 2006; Ryu 2015) and *kipeun-mat* are considered the most important ones and are often referred to as the third taste. *Siwonhan-mat* is a refreshing and pleasurable compounded taste experienced through taste buds and body organs, and includes the sensation of food touching soft tissues in the mouth, swallowing food in the throat, and digestion in the stomach (Kang et al. 2016; Kwon et al. 2017a; Kwon and Chung 2018). *Kipeun-mat* is another important taste in *baro-keumat*, especially in fermented foods such as *makeoli* (Korea traditionally wine), *doenjang, kanjang, kochujang*, and *jangat-ji*, it is also called *kemi* in the Cholla Province in Korea like the taste in *kokumi* in Japan. The sparkling taste in well-fermented *skate* (*hong-eo*) in Cholla-*namdo* is well known as *kemi* due its *kipeun-mat* (Kim 1996; Kim and Jang 2015).

Despite the importance of food culture currently, there is a lack of funding for research on the tastes of Korean food beyond the five basic tastes. A scientific and systematic evaluation of the tastes found in Korean food is needed to develop and improve the exposure of Korean traditional food in the global context.

4.6.3 Siwonhan-mat: *The Third Taste of Korean Foods*

4.6.3.1 Understanding Siwonhan-mat *from Linguistic and Literary Approaches*
4.6.3.1.1 Origin of Siwonhada *(infinitive form of* siwonhan*)* When Koreans talk about the delicious taste of food, the most common word is *siwonhada*. Thus, many non-Koreans who taste Korean foods ask what is the meaning of *siwonhada*. According to the *National Korean Language Dictionary* (Hangeulhakhoe 1991), the usage of *siwonhada* includes: "The weather is refreshing," "The broth of this *kuk* (soup) feels good for digestibility," "I am relieved of my worries," and "He is merry and cheerful, affable and amiable, and clean and neat."

This demonstrates *siwonhada*'s wide use of describing combinations of mind and work; words and behavior; and words related to the body, food, and space (Song 2011). The diverse usage of *siwonhada* suggests that it conveys more than just a mere description of temperature. For example, when someone says the *kuk-mul* (broth of *kuk*) is *siwonhada*, it describes the experience of having hot broth calming the stomach. It does not describe the surface temperature of the broth, but the sensation resulting from consuming the food. *Kuk* with fermented kimchi or dried pollack with *kan* are also dishes described with *siwonhada*. As described previously, *kan* means balancing the salt concentration to enhance the flavor of food (Song 2009; Jang et al. 2016; Kwon et al. 2017a; Kwon 2020). The most common seasoning in Korean cuisine is *kanjang*. Salt and *doenjang* are also widely used (Kwon 2022). In this case, *siwonhada* is used to represent the refreshing sensation experienced during digestion as well. When explaining low temperatures with food, *chagapda* (cool) is used instead of *siwonhada*.

Starting in the 15th century, *siwonhada* began being used in diverse contexts to describe a refreshing and pleasurable sensation (Song 2009). Starting in the late 19th century, *siwonhada* started being used in association with food when quenching thirst with liquids such as water or broth (Song 2011), and when describing low-temperature food. Moreover, cathartic emotions from stories, novels, or movies are often described as *siwonhada* as well. These references suggest that the linguistic origin of *siwonhada* is "being relieved of worries" (Hangeulhakhoe 1991). Also, *siwonhada* means that it is pleasant and vital when cool and refreshing air is inhaled and a hot bath makes our body reboost energy (*qi*). Therefore, *siwonhan-mat* refers to the refreshing and soothing tastes of food regardless of its temperature.

People who are not familiar with the origin of *siwonhada* and non-Korean speakers often perceive the meaning of the word as "cool" and raise questions about the usage of *siwonhada* when eating hot *kuk*. When entering a bath, Koreans (generally adults) often describe the feeling as *siwonhada*. It is a hard concept to grasp for children who often perceive *siwonhada* as cool or cold. As a result, *siwonhada* is frequently perceived as cool, or another antonym of hot. Some scholars have tried to explain this misunderstanding through the concept of polysemy (Lee 2011), viewing *siwonhada* only as a temperature-related word.

In addition, the incorrect translation of Korean words also contributes to the misunderstanding of the word's meaning. For example, *maepda* (spicy) and *siwonhada* are often translated into hot- and cool-temperature-related words. The erroneous meaning of *siwonhada* would spread this way due to mistranslation. Therefore, it would be desirable to retain the original concept of *siwonhada* rather than translating the word as "cool."

4.6.3.1.2 Understanding Siwonhan-mat *from a Scientific Approach* According to the evolutionary point of view, the development of the sense of taste is closely related with human survival instincts (Lee et al. 2013; Ryu 2015). For example, the sense of taste would have been an important determining factor when consuming new food substances in an earlier primitive age. According to the physiological definition of taste as a chemical reaction experienced through taste buds, taste can be split into five basic categories: sweetness, sourness, saltiness, bitterness, and umami (Bear et al. 2006; Ryu 2015). More recently, research has revealed the existence of thermoreceptors, sensory receptors responsible for the sense of pain and temperature. Thermoreceptors react to various temperature levels. However, extremely high or low temperatures activate not only thermoreceptors but also pain receptors, which results in a simultaneous sensation of temperature and pain (Bear et al. 2006). TRPV1, also known as the capsaicin receptor, is the first isolated thermoreceptor and is activated by temperatures greater than 42 °C and the chemical compound found in hot chili peppers, capsaicin (Pingle et al. 2007). Capsaicin of chili is the main element in fermenting kimchi and the red color of chili is the main essence of appetizing taste of Korean food. TRPM8 is activated by temperatures lower than 25 °C (Mckemy 2011). Examples of tastes sensed through thermoreceptors are spiciness, astringency, and temperature-related tastes such as hot and cool.

Historically, Koreans have tried to describe the characteristics of food through a health lens (Anonymous BC 200; Kim et al. 2012) with four attributes (Anonymous 500 BC; Kim et al. 2012). In Korea and China, medicinal and food ingredients are categorized by the four attributes (*qi*) or natures. The four medicinal natures are cold, hot, warm, and cool.

For example, warming ingredients decrease oxygen consumption and slow metabolic activity in the body. In addition, they hinder fluid intake and suppress the central nervous system. Warming ingredients also have anti-inflammatory properties and have the effect of raising yang (*qi*) and warming the body by improving circulation and dispelling cold. On the other hand, cooling ingredients increase oxygen consumption and metabolism. They also promote fluid intake and stimulate the central nervous system. In addition, cooling ingredients have nourishing and detoxifying effects on the blood (Anonymous 500 BC; Kim et al. 2012). In other words, Korean food and its food culture are deeply related to survival and to live and can be conceptualized by the idea of *yaksikdongwon* (medicine and food arises from the same source). About 2,500 years ago, Hippocrates recognized that food was as important as medicine in humans by saying, "Let food be thy medicine and medicine be thy food." Similarly, in Asia, the importance of food in life is acknowledged with the expression *Yaksikdongwon* (a long time ago) (Chung et al. 2016a).

The meaning of *siwonhan-mat* can be properly understood in the context of health and survival, rather than the mere appreciation of smell, color, and taste. *Siwonhan-mat* characterizes Korean food and is a vital concept to understand in Korean food culture.

4.6.3.2 Determining Factors of Siwonhan-mat   As mentioned previously, *siwonhan-mat* is a refreshing taste that is associated with the sensation of food touching soft tissues in the mouth, swallowing food in the throat, and digestion in the stomach. An antonym of *siwonhan-mat* is not *tatheuthan-mat*, but *neukihan-mat*, which describes an unpleasant indigestive feeling.

It is presumed that *siwonhan-mat* is composed of several elements other than the five basic tastes, such as salinity, acidity, spiciness, and a feeling of refreshment. For example, *siwonhan-mat* is often experienced through *kuk* or *tang* (Kwon et al. 2015), types of Korean dishes with broth, and in this case, *siwonhan-mat* is associated with the proper *kan* (Song 2009) of the dish. More research on determining the exact elements of *siwonhan-mat* should be conducted to allow further understanding of this taste. *Kuk* is often mistranslated as "soup." Korean *kuk* is not the same as Western soup, which is served before the main dish rather than with the main dish like *kuk*. *Kuk* helps with digestion when rice is served; they go together like Coke and hamburgers.

4.7 Representative Korean Foods (K-Foods)

As shown in Table 4.1, there are hundred of kinds of Korean foods (K-foods), while there are dozens of representative *bapsang* (K-diet) (Kwon et al. 2017a). Among them, some representative K-foods listed by red letters in Table 4.1 are introduced as follows:

4.7.1 Jang

Jang is the main sauce of Korean foods; *doenjang, kanjang, kochujang*, and *chongkukjang*, are typical fermented soybean products in Korea (Kwon et al. 2015; Kwon 2022; Shin and Jeong 2015). Traditional *jang* (*doenjang* and *kanjang*) is made by making *meju* (looks like brick) using boiled soybean. *Meju* is fermented first with rice straw as a starter culture, which was used to hang up *meju* under the ceiling of thatched-roof house for drying. This dried and surface fermented *meju* is further fermented in brine (salt + water) (Yang et al. 2011). The fermented liquid part (*kanjang*) is separated from the fermented paste (*doenjang*) after fermentation (Park and Park 2018). *Chongkukjang* is short-term fermented foods with cooked soybean for 2–3 days (Chung et al. 2019). *Kochujang* is made mainly from *meju* powder (fermented soybean powder), including red chili powder and small amounts of rice cereal starch (Kwon et al. 2015; Shin and Jeong 2015). These *jangs* have a long history and are the most basic K-foods of Korea and are very healthy foods (Park and Park 2018), because the origin of soybean is Manchuria, where ancient Koreans live.

4.7.2 Yangnyom

Yangnyom is another typical Korean seasoning. In general, ancient people, especially women think about how to eat food deliciously based on taste. Main foodstuffs of Korean food are vegetables, so Korean women found how to eat these vegetables deliciously. Usually if food is cooked with high temperature heating, the food is tasty. But they could not cook vegetables with a high temperature. Vegetables such as kimchi are representative of non-heated cooking, and *namul* is representative low-heated blanched cooking (Kim et al. 2020). To eat fresh or blanched vegetables as delicious food, Koreans developed many yangnyom (sauce for vegetables) using spices such as red pepper, onion, ginger, green onion, and garlic. Korean people usually use red pepper as it is a vibrant red color and deliciously spicy. These *yangnyom* are prepared using *kanjang, doenjang, kochujang*, and sesame and perilla oil (Na and Surh 2018). The main components of the *yangnyom* such as capsaicin, gingerol, allicin, and others are powerful anti-oxidants and anti-inflammatory compounds.

4.7.3 Namul

Namul means all kinds of edible vegetables from mountains and fields as well as *banchan* (Table 4.1) prepared with *namul* (Kim et al. 2020). Among *namul*, wild greens are called *pusae*, while cultivated greens are called *namsae* (National Institute of Korean Language 2017). The Korean vegetable dish *namul* is prepared as fresh (*saengchae*), cooked by blanching, or stir-frying with small amount of oil (*sukchae*) with various seasonings such as *jang* and *yangnyom*. Dried *namul* are first soaked in water, blanched, and then dried. Dried *namul* (bracken, mushroom, eggplant, squash, cucumber, dried radish greens, and aster) is preserved from the past year's harvest to be consumed in the winter (Lee 2018).

4.7.4 Kimchi

Kimchi is a unique and famous fermented food in Korea. Kimchi is the product found accidently from prepared vegetables with *yang-nyom* (Kwon 2019). Usually, it is prepared vegetables with various *yangnyom*, but Koreans could not eat them all. So, they left remaining in the house, and then tasted it couple days later. It was still comfortable and tasty to eat without digestive problems, regardless of unsweet smells. Thus, kimchi is fermented vegetable food with *yangnyom* in Korea, where fermentation of salted vegetables with red chili powder was used as a food preservation method about 2,000–3,000 years ago (Jang et al. 2015, Yang et al. 2015).

There are hundreds of kinds of kimchi in Korea, depending on the raw materials, manufacturing methods, and other characteristics. *Baechu* kimchi mainly prepared with *baechu* cabbage is the major kimchi. These days, the health effects of kimchi in terms of metabolites and microbiomes resulting from fermentation have been scientifically investigated (Park and Ju 2018).

4.7.5 Korean Chili (Korean Red Pepper)

Also, the taste of food is related to the color of food; if we look at the well-cooked food with red color, our saliva increases before eating. Usually Koreans make and cook foods to be delicious with colorful sauces such as red chili powder and red pepper; this is very common in K-food. Korean chili (Korean red pepper) evolved and originated in Korea for half a million years, while chili emerged on earth 19.6 million years ago (Kwon et al. 2017b; Yang et al. 2017). It is not known scientifically in which continent chili initially emerged. However, chili spread into other continents through birds for 10 million years and then evolved to more than 50 different species. Korean chili (*Capsicum annuum*) is unique due to its less spicy and sweet taste, which is quite different from those of Central America and South Asia. Over thousands of years, Koreans found that *baechu* cabbage with red pepper powder for taste could be still edible for 2–3 days without even an odorous smell (Kwon 2019). Therefore, they found very delicious, fermented kimchi.

4.7.6 Jeotgal

Jeotgal is traditional fermented fish food in Korea, produced from the whole meat and/or internal organs of fish and shellfish. Fish and shellfish are highly perishable due to the high moisture content and nutritive elements; thus, *jeotgal* has been produced using salt and fermentation to avoid deterioration from spoilage, autolysis, and microbial activities and to enhance the preservation. *Jeotgal* is an important part of Korean cuisine because of its nutritional value, healthful effects on digestion and appetite, and beneficial microorganisms (Koo and Kim 2018).

4.7.7 Okokbap

Usually, in *Jeongwol Daeboreum* (first full moon in lunar year), cooked *okokbap* (boiled rice with five grains: glutinous rice, red beans, sorghum, and millet) is eaten to celebrate the festival and to pray that all people will be happy and healthy. *Okokbap* are rich in nutrients and healthy due their ingredients. In *Jeongwol Daeboreum*, people believed that they will be rich if they have *okokbap* from three different houses (Han 2005).

4.7.8 Red Bean Juk (Danpat-juk)

Koreans usually make *juk* (like as porridge) using rice, pumpkin, mung bean, and red bean in a year (Han 2005). Especially on *dongji* (winter solstice day), *danpat* (red bean)-*juk* was eaten in the belief that the red color of the beans (azuki beans) had a positive energy that could drive away evil spirits. Azuki beans are rich in nutrients and in addition, and cooked red beans were used to make popular *patbingsu* (shaved ice dessert).

4.7.9 Bibimbap

Bibimbap is rice with mixed meat and assorted vegetables, which has characteristics differing from usual Korean *bapsang* as a meal (Cha 2018; Chung et al. 2015). Westerners often serve a single dish during a meal and bibimbap resembles that, which has made it very favored and loved. It is served as a bowl of warm white rice topped with *namul* (sauteed and seasoned vegetables). Each customer does *bibida* (action of lubrication and mixing with spoon) by himself with the help of *kochujang* and sesame oil in their own bowl (Kwon et al. 2015). Bibimbap is one of the definitive Korean dishes in the eyes of both Koreans and international enthusiasts (Yang et al. 2015). *Jeonju* bibimbap is historical and the most popular bibimbap in Korea as well as in the world.

4.7.10 Doenjang-kuk

Kuk is the second important food in the Korean diet, as shown in Figure 4.1. *Kuk* is essential in Korean *bapsang*. *Doenjang-kuk* is very common, because they can make any kind of *doenjang-kuk* with various substances such as vegetables, seafood, and meat. Spinach, scallion, a curled mallow, and *siraeki* (dried radish greens) are typical substances for vegetable *doenjang-kuk*. Healthy *doenjang* has nutritious vegetables rich in phytochemicals and vitamins and makes food delicious. Epidemiological case data of centenarians of the KuKokSoonDam (Kurye-Koksong-Soonchang-Damyang Province) area of Chollado showed that *doenjang-kuk* is critical for longevity (Kang et al. 2008; Lee 2019).

4.7.11 Miyok-kuk

There are dozens of *kuk* in Korean diet, but *miyok-guk* (sea mustard soup) is very special, because it is a symbol of birthdays for Koreans. By custom, it is the first meal mothers eat after giving birth, so it has become a food representing birth. Even those who dislike *miyok-guk* usually eat it on their birthdays. This *kuk*, which is known as the first *kuk*, is clear and seasoned only with soy sauce and sesame oil, as opposed to ordinary *miyok-kuk* that contains beef. Rich in calcium and iodine, *miyok* helps the womb contract and stimulates the production of new blood cells, whose benefit was first proven scientifically (Korean Food Storytelling 2019).

4.7.12 Sundae and sundae-kuk

Sundae is a type of blood sausage in Korean foods using pork colon (Kwon et al. 2017a; Kwon 2020). Traditional *sundae* is one where pig intestine (colon) is stuffed with *seonji* (blood), minced meats, rice, and vegetables such as green onion and leek, and was an indulgent food consumed during special occasions, festivities, and large family gatherings (Kim and Jang 2014). After the Korean War, when meat was scarce during the period of post-war poverty, artificial edible film and *dangmyeon* replaced intestine and meat fillings in South Korea. Korean *sundae* has their own and long history back to the Kochosun, simultaneously and naturally, they imagine how to eat pork or beef intestine deliciously and safely and developed their own style (Yook 2017). *Sundae-kuk* is another favorite dish as one-bowl food, which is made by adding *sundae* and some other small intestine and boiled.

4.7.13 Kimchi-chigae

Kimchi is always served in Korean *bapsang* (Kwon et al. 2017a). Koreans were so diligent and clever to create more delicious foods using kimchi; kimchi-*kuk*, kimchi-*jeon*, kimchi-*jeonkol*, and kimchi-*chigae*. Kimchi-*chigae* is cooked by putting some chopped *baechu* kimchi and some pork in a pot and boiling them with other *yang-nyom*. There is nothing like a bowl of hot kimchi-*chigae* to be *siwonhan-mat* and relieve stress and anxiety (Lee 2011). It is also the most frequently served dish in Korean homes, perhaps because kimchi is always available in any household throughout the year, and anyone can make a savory *chigae* with well-fermented kimchi alone.

4.7.14 Japchae

A dish that is always served at Korean parties and special occasions is *japche*. The name of *japchae* is a combination of *jap* meaning "miscellaneous and together" and *chae* meaning "vegetables," and thus *japchae* literally means "a mixture of vegetables" (Yoon 2018). The main idea is to combine noodles (*dangmyon*, glass noodle made from sweet potato starch) with *namul* (Kwon et al. 2017a). The components of *namul* are spinach, carrot, onion, and mushroom. Marinated beef strip is also added for individual taste.

4.7.15 Kalbi and Kalbi-chim

Kalbi is a meat dish that is cooked on a grill over charcoal fire by cooking seasoned ribs. It is one of the favorite but expensive cuisines in Korea. The meaning of *kalbi* is ribs of meat. Basically, *kalbi* is from beef ribs, but now sometimes *kalbi* is made using pork ribs because of the price of beef. *Kalbi* is most expensive menu item in Korean restaurants.

Kalbi-chim is cooked by adding a variety of seasonings to carefully prepared beef ribs in a pot, which is then slowly brought to a boil over low heat just to braise some *yangnyom* to be absorbed. *Kalbi-chim* is loved by all, not just because it is nutritious food, high in protein, but also because of its soft texture and rich flavor (Lee 2010b).

4.7.16 Bulgoki *(Grilled seasoned beef)*

Bulgoki is another typical and unique Korean food, which is the meat grilled after seasoning with *yangnyom*. Sliced beef sirloin was used as a meat. Grilling is done just before eating after *yangnyom* is thoroughly absorbed into the meat (Lee 2010b). Once the seasoned beef strips are placed on a shallow grill or pan, the juices from the meat mix, creating a tasty gravy that hugs the meat (Yoon 2018).

4.7.17 Samkyopsal-gui

The most popular menu since 1980 among Korean people who love to grill meat on the table is *samkyopsal-gui*. The meat is called *samkyopsal* (literally meaning "three-layered meats") because it has alternating layers of meat and fat. Basically, roasting the high fat meat at a high temperature caused it to be delicious, and even more with garlic and green chilies (Lee 2011). Usually, they love *samkyopsal* by wrapping lettuce or sesame leaves using sesame oil sauce or *doenjang* (*doenjang* is specially called *ssamjang*).

4.7.18 Jangat-ji

Jangat-ji (pickled vegetables) is the best dish created with *jang*. The original meaning of *jangat-ji* is the fermented *ji* (kimchi) in the *jang* like as *doenjang* and *kochujang* (Yang et al. 2015). Some vegetables or fruits are preserved and aged in *jang*. Numerous ingredients can be used in *jangat-ji*. From radishes, bamboo shoots, dried yellow croaker, garlic or garlic stems, and cucumber in the spring to wild sesame/perilla leaves, green chili, *deodok* (roots of *Codonopsis lanceolata*), bellflower root, plum, persimmon, and winter gourd, all kinds of produce are made into *jangat-ji* at various times of the year (Lee 2010b).

4.7.19 Theokboki

Theok is a Korean traditional valuable cake based on cooked rice. For someone's birthday ceremony or in *Sollal* (lunar new year) and *Chusok* (thanksgiving full moon), Koreans prepared various kinds of *theok* for celebration (Kwon et al. 2017a). After the celebration, *theok* is easily retrograded because of the starch of rice. If one wants to eat *theok* later, it is hard to eat without re-gelatinization by heating like steaming and baking or stir-frying. Baked *theok* (origin of *theok-boki*) was made by heating in the classical brazier, and then eaten by taking a dip of honey or *jochong*, and *kanjang* or *kochujang*. This *theok-boki* was commercialized after the import of wheat flour in 1960 by making cheaper wheat-based *theok*. This *theok-boki* is a Korean favorite, especially *kochujang theok-boki*, coated with mouth-watering *kochujang*, is one of the popular street foods of Korea (Lee 2010b).

4.7.20 Haemul-pajeon

Jeon is a dish made by lightly coating meat, fish, or vegetables with flour and batter, and then shallow frying with sesame or perilla oil on a griddle (Yoon 2018). In the rural area, every sunny day they must work in the farming fields; however, they cannot do any work outside if it rains suddenly. Inevitably, they stay inside the house together, and they think about what food they can prepare easily as munchies between the main meals. *Pa* (green onion) and leek are used as vegetables for making *jeon* because these are always available in the fields, even in a rainy summer. With this historical memory, although they lived in urban areas, having moved from rural areas, they crave a *pajeon* on a rainy day (Kwon et al. 2017b). The delicious *pa* and abundant *haemul* (seafood) blended perfectly to create a savory flavor for *haemul-pajeon*, which quickly became a popular dish throughout the nation (Lee 2010a,b).

4.7.21 Sikhye

Sikhye is a traditional dessert beverage made by fermenting rice in malt (*yot-kireum*). Also known as sweet liquor (*kamju*), it is called *sikhye* if you drink it together with the grains and *kamju* when the liquor is separated out. *Sikhye*'s essential ingredient is malt made from sprouted barley. Since malt is rich in amylase, a diastatic enzyme, *sikhye* has been traditionally offered as dessert drink after eating heavy meals on celebration or festival days. It was a favorite digestive tonic after overindulging during the days when other forms of digestive aids were not readily available (Kwon et al. 2017a; Korean Food Storytelling 2019).

4.7.22 Sungnyung

In Korea, people drink *sungnyung* (like tea) to finish off a meal (Moose 1911). It is a traditional Korean drink made from *nurungji* (leftover scotched rice crust) that forms on the bottom of a pot after cooking rice. Water is poured on this brown crust and the contents are put to a simmer until the water gains enough flavor of the scorched rice. *Sungnyung* helps in digestion and is good to comfort the stomach and feel happy.

Conclusions

In the age of globalization and international engagement, many non-Koreans are very much interested in Korean foods and diet because of its history, ethnicity, and healthiness. This chapter answers the question: What is the nature of the Korean diet in addition to history, culture, and health? The values of the K-diet are respect and consideration, harmony and balance, and healthiness. When defining the K-diet, various components are considered, such as raw materials or ingredients, traditional cooking methods, technology, and fundamental principles and knowledge. However, it would be preferable to establish the definition of Korean food by focusing on the preservation of traditional methods and core principles. The Korean meal table (*bapsang*) is characterized by servings of *bap*, *kuk*, and *banchan* on one table. The K-diet is composed of *bap* and *kuk*, and various *banchans* with one serving called *bapsang*. Kimchi is always served at every meal. While various cooking methods are used in Korean cuisine, the most representative method is fermentation, which enhances both the taste and preservation of the food. The principal aspects of the K-diet include proportionally high consumption of vegetables (*namul*), moderate to high consumption of legumes and fish, and low consumption of red meat. *Banchan* is mostly seasoned with various *jang* (fermented soy products), and *yangnyom* with medicinal herbs, and sesame or perilla oil. The points of taste in a K-diet are quite different from those of Western tastes.

Unique expressions of Korean taste are *kan*, the right taste (*baro-keumat*), and *siwonhan-mat*, which is typical in Korean delicious tastes. In Korean cuisine, *doenjang*, *kanjang*, and salt are commonly used seasonings. A couple of representative *bapsangs* and some representative K-foods from among hundreds of kinds of Korean foods were described. Overall, this chapter provided very important perspectives in making these diverse connections for those learning about Korean food. Moreover, this is vital to promote the cultural values of Korea (K-value) by bringing together traditional principles and scientific evidence.

Acknowledgments

This work is done with the support of the project of nutritional epigenomics study on a Korean healthy diet (E0150300-05) in part from the Korea Food Research Institute. I would like to thank Soon Hee Kim, Myung Sunny Kim, Hye Jeong Yang, Min Jung Kim, and Dae Ja Jang from the Korea Food Research Institute. I also thank Professor Oran Kwon from Ewha University for the kind comments.

References

Adamsson V, Reumark A, Cederholm T, Vessby B, Riserus U and Johansson G (2012) What is a healthy Nordic diet? Foods and nutrients in the nordiet study. *Food Nutrition Research* 56.1 (2012) DOI: 10.3402/fnr.v56i0.18189

Anonymous. (BC 200?) New-nongbonchokyung. China.

Anonymous. (BC 500?) Hwangje-naekyung. China.

Bear MF, Connors BW and Paradiso MA (2006) *Neuroscience: Exploring the Brain*. Philadelphia, PA, USA: Lippincott Williams and Wilkins.

Cha YS (2018) Bibimbap as a Balanced One-Dish Meal, in *Korean Functional Foods: Composition, Processing and Health Benefits* (edited by Park KY, Kwon DY, Lee KW, and Park S). pp. 421–439. New York, NY, USA: CRC Press.

Choi HS (2009) *All Human Senses*, Seoul, Korea.

Chung HK (2015) The meaning and symbolism of Korean food culture. *Asia Review* 5:97–121.

Chung KR, Yang HJ, Jang DJ and Kwon DY (2015) Historical and biological aspects of bibimbap, a Korean ethnic food. *Journal Ethnic Foods* 2:74–83.

Chung HK, Chung KR and Kim HJ (2016a) Understanding Korean food culture from paintings. *Journal Ethnic Foods* 3:42–50.

Chung HK, Yang HJ, Shin D and Chung KR (2016b) Aesthetics of Korean foods: the symbol of Korean culture. *Journal Ethnic Foods* 3:178–188.

Chung KR, Jang DJ and Kwon DY (2019) The history and science of chongkukjang, a Korean fermented soybean product. *Journal Ethnic Foods* 7:6:5 10.1186/s42779-019-0004-8

Ferrieres J (2004) The French paradox: lessons for other countries. *Heart* 90:107–111.

Hangeulhakhoe (1991) *Grand Dictionary of Hangeul Seoul.* Korea.

Han YS (2005) *Invitation to Korean Cuisine.* Seoul, Korea: Sookmyung Women's Uiversity Press.

Health Magazine (2006) *World's Five Healthiest Foods,* March Issue, Health Magazine.

Hur J (1610) *Donguibogam.* Korea.

Hwang HS, Han BR and Han BJ (2005) *Korean Traditional Foods.* Seoul, Korea: Kyomunsa.

Jang DJ, Chung KR, Yang HJ, Kim KS and Kwon DY (2015) Discussion on the origin of kimchi, representative of Korean unique fermented vegetables. *Journal Ethnic Foods* 2:126–136.

Jang DJ, Lee AJ, Kang SA, Lee SM and Kwon DY (2016) Does siwonhan-mat represent delicious in Korean foods? *Journal Ethnic Foods* 3:159–162.

Kang IH Suh KD, Cho HL, Lee JS, Yang SJ, Park MS, Park SC, Yang DS, Pes GM, Salaris L, Kazuhiko T, Tomoaki K, Park SC, Chun KS, Choi SJ, Corriga A, Lee MS, Kim HD, Kwak CS and Oh SI (2008) Declarartion of Sunchang 'Longevity Community', Sunchang, Chollabuk-do, Korea.

Kang SA, Oh HJ, Jang DJ, Kim MJ and Kwon DY (2016) Siwonhan-mat: the third taste of Korean foods. *Journal Ethnic Foods* 3:61–68.

Kim CG (2008) A study on meaning of the taste adjective. *Eomunhak* 100:1–30.

Kim JS (1996) *Exploring the Namdo Foods and Their Culture.* Seoul, Korea: Kyung Hyang News, January 25th.

Kim K, Park S, Yang M and Choi Y (2012) *Siklyobonchohak, Eosongdang.* Korea.

Kim SH and Jang DJ (2015) *Fabulous Korean Ethnic Foods, Namdo.* Seoul, Korea: Elsevier Korea.

Kim SH, Kim MS, Lee MS, Park YS, Lee HJ, Kang S, Lee HS, Lee KF, Yang HJ, Kim MJ, Lee Y-E and Kwon DY (2016) Korean diet (K-diet): Characteristics and historical background. *Journal Ethnic Foods* 3:26–31.

Kim YHB and Jang A (2014) Ethnic meat products: Japan and Korea, in *Encyclopedia of Meat Sciences* (edited by Dikeman M and Devine C), 2nd, pp. 543–549. San Diego, CA, USA: Academic Press.

Kim SH, Kwon DY and Shin D (2020) Namul, driving force behind health and vegetables consumption in Korea. *Journal of Ethnic Foods* 7:15.

Ko BS, Park S and Chung KJ (2014) *Korean Traditional Medicine and Nutrition*. Daejeon, Korea: Korea Institute of Oriental Medicine (in Korean).

Koo OK and Kim YM (2018) Jeotgal (Fermented Fish): Secret of Korean Seasonings. In *Korean Functional Foods: Composition, Processing and Health Benefits* (edited by Park KY, Kwon DY, Lee KW and Park S), pp. 183–215. New York, NY, USA: CRC Press.

Korean Food Storytelling (2019) https://www.hansik.org/en/board.do?cmd=list&bbs_id=211&menu=PEN3020000&lang=en. Assessed 13 Mar 2019).

Kwon DY (2015) Why ethnic foods? *Journal Ethnic Foods* 2:91.

Kwon DY (2016) Seoul declaration of Korean diet. *Journal Ethnic Foods* 3:1–4.

Kwon DY (2017a) Ethnic foods and their taste: salt and sugar. *Journal Ethnic Foods* 4:133–134.

Kwon DY (2017b) Why they crave pajeon in rainy days, Food Oesik Kyongje. July 17th, Seoul, Korea (in Korea).

Kwon DY (2018) Lifestyle and health in post-industrial era. *Annals Nutrition Food Sci.* 2:1–2.

Kwon DY (2019) Humanities of Korean Food, Health Letters, Seoul, Korea (in Korean).

Kwon DY (2019) The answer is in Korean traditional bapsang. In *Health Centanarian: Story of Health Foods*. pp. 220–286. Sikanyon, Seoul, Korea: Sikanyon Publisher (in Korean).

Kwon DY (2020) Diet in Korea. In *Handbook of Eating and Drinking* (editied by Herbert LM), pp. 1435–1466. Switzland: Springer.

Kwon DY (2022) Jang and Korean Food Culture. In *Overview of Korean Jang (Fermented Soybean Products) and Manufacturing* (edited by Shin DH, Kwon DY, Jeong DY and Nam YK). pp. 33–62, Korea Jang Cooperative Association, Seoul, Korea.

Kwon DY and Chung KR (2018) Korean diets and their tastes. In *Korean Functional Foods: Composition, Processing and Health Benefits* (edited by Park KY, Kwon DY, Lee KW and Park S). pp. 23–42, CRC Press, New York, NY, USA.

Kwon DY, Jang DJ, Yang HJ and Chung KR (2014) History of Korean *gochu, gochujang*, and kimchi. *Journal Ethnic Foods* 1:3–7.

Kwon DY, Chung KR, Yang HJ and Jang DJ (2015) Gochujang (Korean red pepper paste): A Korean ethnic sauce, its role and history. *Journal Ethnic Foods* 2:29–35.

Kwon DY, Lee YE, Kim MS, Kim SH et al. (2017a) *What is Korean Diet: History, Culture and Health*. Seoul, Korea: Korea Food Research Institute (in Korean).

Kwon DY, Chung KR and Yang HJ (2017b) *The Truth of Birth and Propogation of Chili (Korean Red Pepper)*. Seoul, Korea: Free Academy (in Korean).

Lee KS (2010a) *Korean Food, The Originality: Becoming one with the Universe; Communication and Harmonization with Nature*. Seoul, Korea: Donga-ilbo.

Lee KS (2010b) *Korean Food, The Impression: Mixing, Wrapping, and Immersing; Meddling Food Together.* Seoul, Korea: Donga-ilbo.

Lee MS (2019) What do Korean centanarian in longevity area eat? In *Health Centanarian: Story of Health Foods.* pp. 53–77. Seoul, Korea: Sikanyon (in Korean).

Lee SY (2011) A study on contronymy in Korean. *J Korean Linguistics* 61:265–289.

Lee YE (2018) Namul, Korean Vegetable Dishes. In *Korean Functional Foods: Composition, Processing and Health Benefits* (edited by Park KY, Kwon DY, Lee KW and Park S), pp. 385–419. New York, NY, USA: CRC Press.

Lee J, Jeong S, Rho JO and Park K (2013) A study of adjectives for sensory evaluation of taste in Korea language. *Science Emotion Sensibility* 16.

Li X, Staszewski L, Xu H, Durick K, Zoller M and Adler E (2002) Human receptors for sweet and umami taste. *Proceedings of the National Academy of Sciences of the United States of America* 99:4692–4696.

Mckemy DD (2011) A spicy family tree: TRPV1 and its thermoceptive and nociceptive lineage. *The EMBO Journal* 30:453–455.

Moose JR (1911) *Village Life in Korea.* Nashville, TN: House of ME Church.

Na HK and Surh YJ (2018) Yangnyom (Spices) and Health Benefits. In *Korean Functional Foods: Composition, Processing and Health Benefits* (edited by Park KY, Kwon DY, Lee KW and Park S), pp. 257–290. New York, NY, USA: CRC Press.

National Institute of Korean Language (2017) Standard Korean Dictionary. http://staweb2.korean.go.kr/search/List-dic.jsp. Accessed 14 May 2017.

Park KY and Ju J (2018) Kimchi and Its Health Benefits. In *Korean Functional Foods: Composition, Processing and Health Benefits* (edited by Park KY, Kwon DY, Lee KW and Park S), pp. 43–77. New York, NY, USA: CRC Press.

Park J and Kwock CK (2015) Sodium intake and prevalence of hypertension, coronary heart disease, and stroke in Korean adults. *Journal Ethnic Foods* 2:92–96.

Park KY and Park ES (2018) Health benefits of Doenjang and Kanjang. In *Korean Functional Foods: Composition, Processing and Health Benefits* (edited by Park KY, Kwon DY, Lee KW and Park S), pp. 43–77. New York, NY, USA: CRC Press.

Pingle SC, Matta JA and Ahern GP (2007) Capsaicin Receptor: TRPV1 A Promiscuous TRP Channel. In *Transient Receptor Potential (TRP) Channels* (edited by Flockerzi V and Nilius B), Handbook of Experimental Pharmacology: Vol 179. Springer, Berlin: Heidelberg. https://doi.org/10.1007/978-3-540-34891-7_9

Ryu MR (2015) *Easy Science Underlying Taste.* Seoul, Korea: Ministry of Science, ICT and Future Planning.

Shin DH and Jeong D (2015) Korean traditional fermented soybean products: *Jang. Journal Ethnic Foods* 2:2–7.

Simini B (2000) Serge Renaud: from French paradox to Cretan miracle. *Lancet* 355:48.

Song HJ and Lee HJ (2014) Consumption of Kimchi, a salt fermented vegetable, is not associated with hypertension prevalence. *Journal Ethnic Foods* 1:8–12.

Song JH (2009) *A Study on the Diachronic Change of Temperature Sensation Words*. PhD Thesis, Kyungbuk University.

Song JH (2011) On an aspect of the meaning change of the 'Siwonhada'. *The Korean Language and Literature* 111:37–56.

Surh YJ (2003) Cancer chemoprevention with dietary phytochemicals. *Nature Review, Cancer* 3:768–780.

Willett WC, Sacks F, Trichopoulou A et al. (1995) Mediterranean diet pyramid: a cultural model for healthy eating. *American Journal Clinical Nutrition* 61:1402S–1406S.

Woo SH (2018) *Origin of Kochosun Civilization and Lyoha Culture, Series of Kochosun Civilization*, Volume 3. Seoul, Korea: Jisik & Industry.

Yang HJ, Park S, Pak V, Chung KR and Kwon DY (2011) Fermented soybean products and their bioactive compounds. In *Soybean and Health* (Edited by El-Shemy H). pp. 21–58. Rijeka, Croatia: Intech.

Yang HJ, Jang DJ, Chung KR, Kim KS and Kwon DY (2015) Origin names of gochu, kimchi, and bibimbap. *Journal Ethnic Foods* 2:162–172.

Yang HJ, Chung KR and Kwon DY (2017) DNA sequence analysis tells the truth of the origin, propagation, and evolution of chili (red pepper). *Journal Ethnic Foods* 4:154–162

Yook KH (2017) *Sundae Silok (Real Story of Sundae)*. Seoul, Korea: BR Media (in Korean).

Yoon JA (2018) K-food: Combining Flavor, Health and Nature. In *Korean Culture*, Series 9. Seoul, Korea: Korean Culture and Information Service, Hansik Foundation.

Yoon SS (1999) *The Culture and History of Korean Foods*. Seoul, Korea: Shinkwang.

5

KOREAN FERMENTED FOODS FOR HEALTHIER LONGEVITY

DONG-HWA SHIN

Emeritus Prof. of Chonbuk National
University. Rep. of Korea

Contents

DOI: 10.1201/9781003275732-6

5.1 Introduction: A Song in Praise of Fermented Foods

It is natural that changes in our lives respond to time and environment in which we live in, which bring many layers of mental and physical challenges for the quality of health and wellness in our lives. This makes us question and reflect on the meaning of life and what it is to live healthy and have long lives with joy and happiness. In this context, the aesthetic sense of slowness is rising in some ways as we get tired of the rapid pace of society and daily lives. This is also extended into our food and diet, in which as opposed to fast food, slow food is slowly being mentioned, and the concept of a slow city emerges where we take time to walk slowly around *Dulle-gil* to look around and look inward at oneself in reflection to connect more widely with nature and life around us. As a result of this thinking and desire, the facilities are being built in various parts of the country to attract tourists. The passage of time is constant, but our mind is in a hurry, and we are buried in a speed war where we have the desire to do more at the same time, produce more, and evaluate only the results of the hour as the best thing as we are in constant competition. While it is important to do many things in our finite lives, we hope that the result of the reflective layering of time will be more precious.

In connection this context, food is no exception as many processed foods are changing quickly and the process is focused on rapid mass production and easily available fast foods to eat, and we live in an age where we cannot wait and are not connected to the diversity of ecology around us. In the current market, various convenient foods such as lunch boxes, *Gimbap* (lapped cooked rice with seaweed), and hamburgers for people who eat solely on such fast foods are growing rapidly and home meal replacement (HMR) is worth three trillion won ($3.5 billion) in the marketplace (Bumedsanpharoke and Ko 2021). They account for a large portion of processed foods in distribution and this trend is not likely to change easily in the future. The most important function of food is to supply nutrients to the body and to maintain vitality, and the next function is to satisfy hunger and to make people feel happy by giving them a feeling of fullness is also important. The euphoria of eating food is thought to be the taste, smell, and texture. Where does the taste and smell come from? It, of course, is based on the ingredients originally contained in the raw materials, but many ingredients are newly made during the cooking or food processing process, and they play an important role. Although different food processes are related to the direct cause that affects the taste of food, in particular, many changes occur due to a heating process that plays a crucial role in softening the food biological tissue to easily eat and improve the flavor to digest well. These are all physical and chemical changes, and in some ways, these are simple processes that do not take much time.

However, in contrast to fast-food concepts, the fermentation process that contributes to changes in flavor, smell, and tissue is completely different. In this slow process, time is given to allow the functions of microorganisms or enzymes from the external environment to operate and function to create the quality and benefits of the targeted foods for our palate and human consumption. In this situation, conditions such as adequate nutrients, temperature, and humidity of natural conditions are required for microorganisms to multiply and operate with harmony, and sufficient process and action is needed to produce the desired product and time is needed to do so. For this reason, fermented foods are also foods where we wait and with reflection allow leisure while we produce and enjoy the food. A representative Korean fermented food, kimchi, takes at least two to three days to several months to get its favorable taste, and fermented soybean products must endure at least two to three months to one year, or a few more years, to enjoy the flavor of its essence. Alcoholic drinks, salted seafood products, and others will give us their distinguished and unique taste and aroma only after a period of wholesome microbial processing.

Fermented foods are made from a process of combination of microorganisms and time, and it is also a process and effort where the best product emerges and surpasses quality towards producing the best masterpieces only when all conditions, such as raw materials, temperature, and humidity, are satisfied. Fermentation goes beyond just the differentiation of quality but gives us many benefits. Fermented foods provide a subtle and deep taste and aroma with the primary role as nourishing food, while several beneficial microorganisms involved in a fermentation process enter our intestines to present various beneficial effects such as obesity control, cholesterol-lowering effect and increasing digestion rate, and synthesis of special healthy ingredients. Luxury soybean products, luxury kimchi, world-famous vinegars, and wine amounting to millions of won a bottle are all rare products made by microorganisms. It is also meaningful to mass produce and sell a lot, but it is time to make one's own branded products and make higher value-added foods in the world and promote the real value of Korea as a principal country for health-targeted family of fermented foods for longevity and quality of life. To achieve this, a comprehensive study is needed to reverse-engineer healthy products with tools of food engineering, biotechnology, nutritional science, fermentation engineering, industrial engineering, packaging technology, and food science integrated together.

5.2 Fermented Foods in Our Daily Lives Came from Early Earth Biology

The debate over how the universe was first created continues with philosophical and scientific interpretations. If we look at the Earth in the universe with a narrow view, the first living thing on this planet, the bacteria (Schopf and Packer 1987), likely evolved about 3.3–3.5 billion years ago, due to the right natural conditions for the first simple cellular life. The bacteria began to use the geothermal resources around them to sustain and multiply and subsequently resulted in diversity of organisms in different ecological niches which then impacted and changed the air composition of the Earth. For a long time, primitive bacteria, including algae, began to produce oxygen-rich air into various compositions on the Earth through enzyme action, nitrogen fixation, and photosynthesis. As life evolved, complex amino acids and vitamins were needed for the survival of these diversified bacteria, and these ingredients were absorbed from different ecological niches. Much before photosynthesis, one of the first revolutionary functions of these life-evolving processes was the ability to transform sugar into energy (Kayhanian et al. 2007). Here, because photosynthesis was yet to evolve, this reaction took place in the water or in the mud under no oxygen or low oxygen conditions, and this biological action began to take effect and has been passed on to metabolic processes we call fermentation until now, hundreds of millions of years later. In the subsequent circumstances the first bacterial photosynthetic life that came later gave rise to oxygen environment that widened the complexity of biology from prokaryotes towards eukaryotes. Yet the fermentation-based bacterial and yeast life still exists with photosynthesis coupled oxygen-based life that is dominant in eukaryotes.

As bacteria evolved into many forms, some had the ability for nitrogen fixation and to create organic nitrogen compounds for all plants, and several other species used carbon dioxide in the air to create photosynthesis, creating a wider base and complexity for major macronutrients such as carbohydrates, proteins, and fats. These primary metabolites produced by the bacteria and other metabolic interconversions of these primary metabolites were the most innovative biological changes in the history of life on Earth. In addition, the oxygen produced in the photosynthesis process of the higher-evolved plants was also responsible for raising the oxygen from the initial 0.0001% to the present 21%. The photosynthetic prokaryotic algae were the earliest life forms to release oxygen and later it was dominated by eukaryotic algae and plants, which used oxygen for energy interconversion and also resulted in non-photosynthetic eukaryotes also doing the same thing. The reason why the oxygen ratio in the atmosphere remains at 21% is complex but is thought to be triggered by the evolution of prokaryotic and eukaryotic photosynthetic life that is the foundation of our macronutrient-dominated food system today. Yet, how fermentation interacts with photosynthetic life to make a wide variety of foods and micronutrients and other bioactive chemicals and support our beneficial microbiome and wider foundation of resilience of biological systems in the diverse ecology of Earth may be the key to healthy, sustainable living and longevity.

5.3 Discovery of Microorganisms and Meaning of Fermentation

For a long time, it was not possible to clearly determine the appearance of bacteria, but fossils allowed us to estimate their shapes and structures. The first person to observe bacteria with the naked eye was the Dutch merchant and scientist, Antonier Philips Van Leeuwenhoek (1632–1723). He used a small single lens to make a 200-fold magnification microscope to observe and record many microbes and confirm their existence. This 200-fold microscope using a small single lens immediately allowed observation of different microbes and to record their diversity. Christian Ehrenberg (1795–1829) renamed the "animalcule" named by Leeuwenhoek as a "bacterium," which means "a club" in Greek. At this time, it was not known that they caused diseases including epidemics such as plagues, but were believed wrongly to be the cause of the disease called miasma, which refers to a poison of physicochemical nature, and there was no recognition of a link of bacterial infection with diseases (Collen 2015).

The foundation of modern microbiology was established by Louis Pasteur (1822–1895) of France and Robert Koch (1843–1910) of Germany. Pasteur proved by experiment that the cause of decomposition was due to microorganisms, and Koch established a pure culture technology of microorganisms using a solid medium. Later, *Bacillus anthracis* (1876), *Mycobacterium tuberculosis* (1882), and *Vibrio cholerae* (1883) were discovered. Since then, the field of microbiology has greatly improved, and after the discovery of microorganisms, there has been large developments that impacted the field of food production and food science. Soon it was discovered that the cause of food spoilage is microorganisms; they are used positively to also make food products such as wine, beer, vinegar, and pickles via fermentation. The microorganisms involved in the fields of food include bacteria, molds, yeasts, and viruses (Shin et al. 2016).

Among important process involved in food spoilage and food product formation is fermentation. Fermentation in a broad sense means "to decompose or transform organic matter by the action of enzymes produced by microorganisms in the absence of oxygen." Since microorganisms first appeared as life on Earth, a fermentation process was used as a means of utilizing the carbon resources around them for survival. The word "fermentation" comes from the Latin word *fervere*, which means "boil," and it was soon after that humans began to recognize the natural phenomenon of fermentation. When grapes or fruits were dropped on the ground, the first fermentation took place by yeasts (it formed bubbles that was like boiling), and honey, which is the first natural sweetener, was diluted with rainwater and that caused fermentation. Thus, the recognition of fermentation began with the fermentation of wine and other liquors, and the fermentation techniques began to be widely used after that. Wine was made at least 10,000 BC and it is estimated that the Egyptians made beer using malt from 5000–6000 BC based on the records on the murals. In the case of bread, one of earliest fermented foods, it is known that bread was made by the Egyptians through kneading flour around 4000 BC. They used the sugars in the dough for raising the dough that is permeated by carbonated gases produced by yeasts.

Fermentation was used as a means of surviving and a breeding process of microorganisms before human beings appeared on this planet, and the process did not change much until the present day. One of the features is that it often does not need oxygen, which is the primordial condition of early Earth, and in only some organisms oxygen is needed to multiply and reproduce itself under some ecological niches. Thus, fermentation was a means of obtaining energy for survival from the early appearance of life on Earth, and various by-products were created in the fermentation process to be used by the other organisms that lived on the succession of metabolic processes. Therefore, the fermentation process is the oldest biological change in nature and is one of the unique natural metabolic phenomena that has continued to be critical across diverse ecologies of creation on Earth and continues to be important for higher forms of life to live sustainably.

Fermentation is closely related to decomposition, which is the same action that is caused by microorganisms, but what is beneficial by human standards is fermentation and it typically happens in the absence of oxygen, and what is not good or may cause harm is called decomposition, which is dependent on an aerobic process. Although these are distinguished by the same concept performed by microorganisms, these are classified according to the usefulness of the final product. For instance, *cheonggukjang* (partially fermented soybean product dominated in later stages by *Bacillus*) is a good decomposition product used by Korean people, but non-Korean cultures who have never seen such products will say it is decomposed or rotten. Figure 5.1 shows a simple description of a fermentation process (Shin 2021).

As shown in Figure 5.1, fermentation is a process of producing enzymes, which are required by microorganisms, on their own and in which these enzymes act on substrate materials to ferment without oxygen or decompose with oxygen to produce various products.

5.4 Products by the Fermentation Process and Applications Associated with Fermentation Technology

Microorganisms have had a profound effect on our lives and health in various fields that are critically essential to our well-being. On the

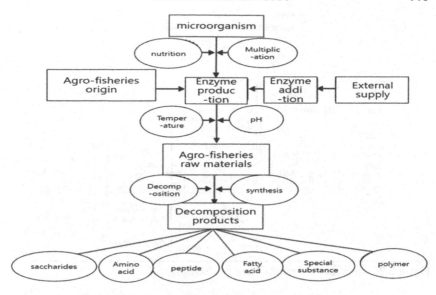

Figure 5.1 Fermentation process performed by microorganisms and enzymes.

negative effect of fermentation, it causes disease or food decomposition, but on the positive side, it creates a diverse array of fermented by-products that enrich our lives and create new materials to enhance functions or enhance it by adding value to our products. It plays an important role in protecting human health in many positive ways while enriching our dining table through producing unique fermented foods. Microorganisms involved in fermentation also have other functions that play a positive role in human health in newly emerging areas of functional foods and microbiome-based health beyond fermentation (Sanath and Nayak 2015; Tamang et al. 2015). The fields of producing fermented products by utilizing microorganisms have been extensively developed. In the case of the industrial fields based on the microorganisms involved in fermentation, a wide range of products and industries have been developed globally. It is applicable to the production of physiologically active substances or food additives, nutrients or new ingredients, and enzymes, starting from a wide array of accessible fermented food sectors and particularly in Asia. Furthermore, these processes can be used for smelting minerals and the biological treatment of industrial or livestock wastewater, which is a problem worldwide, can also be performed using

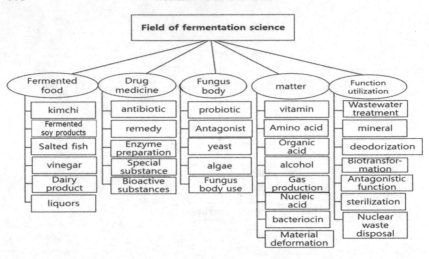

Figure 5.2   Application of fermentation-related technology.

microorganisms. There has also been a theory that nuclear wastes can be disposed of as microorganisms at a low cost in a short period of time. Fermentation technologies are used in a wide range of fields, and each has a different purpose and source of materials or processing technology. The application of fermentation-related technology is presented in Figure 5.2 (Shin 2019).

As shown in Figure 5.2, fermentation technology can be used in many ways and fermented foods belong to one small area of the wide range of possibilities. In terms of industrial scale, food and medicine cover a large portion, but the application of it as food additives as organic acids, and of microorganisms for water treatment, odor removal, and antagonistic microorganisms will also likely be highlighted in future industrialization processes. In addition, studies will be conducted to give many different functions or enhance certain functions through genetic modification or gene editing because microorganisms are amenable to being genetically engineered with exciting new technologies for diverse applications.

5.5 Fermented Foods of Korea

It is reported that there are about 5,000 kinds of fermented foods produced and consumed in many countries around the world. The different kinds of fermented foods used is deeply related to the environmental conditions of diverse ecological niches of humanity and natural sources, the wisdom and history of the inhabitants, and their dietary life. In general, when observing a country with a long history, various fermented foods have appeared over their history and societies are creative in accordance with the time shown in history and their need for a solution when challenged by a need. Looking at fermented foods that are used around the world, we can understand that there are many different items in East and Southeast Asian countries, where grains and vegetables are the main natural resources compared to the West, where meat and wheat are the main staple foods. Fermented foods can be divided into acidity, alkalinity, and others depending on the characteristics of the final product. These depend on the microorganisms concerned and raw materials involved in fermentation. Microorganisms involved in fermentation are mainly bacteria that are involved in the production of the wide range of products, and the variety of microorganisms is very diverse. The representative bacteria in this category are largely lactic acid bacteria and are classified as aerobic, anaerobic, and facultative bacteria depending on oxygen demands. Many dairy products have utilized lactic acid bacteria, and *chunggukjang* of Korea is a soybean product fermented/decomposed by *Bacillus*. Yeast are mainly involved in the production of alcohol-fermented drinks and produce alcohol as the final product. In addition, yeast contributes to soy sauce or other fermented foods, affecting flavors. Next, there are not many related products of molds, but they are often used in products with grain and soybeans for initial aerobic breakdown for subsequent succession by bacteria and yeasts to make desired fermented products. A switch of this process is Korea's *meju* (a block-type soybean product), a representative mold aerobic growth product but with an earlier phase of succession by other microorganisms such as yeast, and Indonesia's *tempe* is also one of the products involved where the final step is an aerobic process and earlier steps may involve fermentation without the need of oxygen, as in the moldy cheese-making process in the West. In general, fermentation by bacteria and yeast is rapid, usually finishing within one to several days, but molds take weeks or months and are dominated by an aerobic process succeeding earlier anaerobic fermentation processing by other microorganisms with *tempe* and moldy cheese being good examples.

When looking at Korean fermented foods more closely, the origin of Korean fermented foods dates to over 2000 years to BC based on various excavated earthenware items. Although these fermented foods may not be the same as the present ones, these are assumed to have changed continuously due to the natural environment and products produced by the Korean people during their lives. It is believed that the idea of how to make a tasteful side dish is different from that of a rice-based diet was the reason for the differentiation of the side dish from the staple food. Vegetables were easily obtained from nature as the main substrate for ingredients of the side dish, but the vegetables themselves do not have any special taste. Thus, fermentation techniques with salt were introduced, which led to the establishment of fermented foods that ensured both taste and long-term storage. For a long time, fermented foods relied on natural conditions. Although there may have been minor differences due to changes in raw materials, there may not have been much difference in basic processes. The fermentation food industry was greatly developed as the technology for managing artificial fermentation processes, which was introduced according to learning as modern technology evolved and developed and with it fermentation with microorganisms was also aligned. The characteristics of Korean fermented foods was easily developed by utilizing all the raw materials produced in this land. Salt was easily obtained from the early days of history because the Korean peninsula is surrounded by the sea on three sides, and most fermented foods were based on salting. Currently, fermented foods that are produced in Korea and consumed largely are kimchi, fermented soybean products, salted fish products (*jeotgal*), and vinegars. These are the four most famous fermented foods in Korea. Alcohol-fermented drinks are classified as favorite alcoholic beverages and excluded from this list.

5.6 Kimchi

Kimchi production and processing mainly uses several kinds of vegetables but it can be mixed with fruits and fish, raw or fermented, including the use of various spices, like red pepper, after being pickled in salt. The growth of putrefactive microorganisms and food poisoning bacteria are inhibited by salting and the lactic acid producing bacteria. The lactic acid bacteria, which are involved in the fermentation, mainly come from raw substrate ingredients such as cabbage, garlic, and red pepper, and they lead to fermentation. Kimchi is mixed with various ingredients in addition to the main ingredients of Korean cabbage and radish, which determine the type and quality of kimchi. The essential ingredient in kimchi is red pepper, which has the most characteristic functions of taste, flavor, and color. In addition, garlic, ginger, chives, and sea staghorn are important ingredients in determining the final quality of kimchi. Currently, there are almost 200 kinds of kimchi surveyed across Republic of Korea, and some people say that the type of kimchi is proportional to the number of Korean housewives, so there is also diversity of preference and taste of the final product.

5.6.1 History of Kimchi

It is not known exactly when Korean traditional kimchi began, but the fact that red pepper is mixed with vegetables to become the present kimchi is deeply related to the traditional history of red peppers. The inflow of red peppers was introduced long before the theory that it came with the Japanese invasion of Korea and some argued that the variety is different from that of other countries (Kwon et al. 2017). The name and chronology of preparing kimchi throughout Korean history is shown in Table 5.1.

Table 5.1 Trend in preparing kimchi based on its name (Choi 2004)

AGE	ANCIENT PERIOD	THREE KINGDOMS	UNIFIED SILLA DYNASTY, GORYEO PERIOD	CHOSEON DYNASTY
Name	醢 (salted fermented fish) 菹 (salted cabbage)	醢 (salted meat) 菹 (salted cabbage)	Ji (漬): salted vegetable Chimchae (浸菜) (Fermented vegetable): Kimchi	Ji (漬): salted vegetable Chimchae (浸菜) (Fermented vegetable): Kimchi
Main raw material	Wild vegetables, cultivated vegetables	Vegetables including radish, eggplant, and pumpkin	Various vegetables	Variable vegetables, white cabbage

As shown in Table 5.1, kimchi represents the trend of raw materials used, and it is believed that Korean cabbage became common during the Choseon Dynasty. Beginning in the Choseon Dynasty, various literature showed different records of diets and foods and it was discovered that various spices were mixed, similar to the kimchi of today during the 1600–1700s. Various records at that time included details of the raw materials used to make kimchi and ways to make kimchi. The cultivation of Korean cabbage dates from the end of the 19th century to the beginning of the 20th century, and its use has increased significantly. The quality Korean cabbage was established in the 1850s.

5.6.2 Industry of Kimchi

Kimchi is the most typical traditional fermented food and represents an annual market of one trillion won. The production reached 438,000 tons (2015) and the output is on the decline every year. This is the result of decreased annual consumption per person, and the main reason is due to the lack of preference for kimchi among the younger generation. Exports of kimchi reached $81,000 for 24,000 tons, but imports amounted to $129,000 for 276,000 tons. It shows that the trade imbalance in kimchi is very serious and may cause concerns that the status of Korea as the kimchi-producing country is faltering.

5.6.3 Kinds of Kimchi and How to Make it

The name of kimchi depends on the main ingredient. The main vegetable substrates are Korean cabbage kimchi, *chonggak* kimchi using radishes, and *kakdugi* with diced radishes. The sub-ingredients are red pepper powder, garlic, green onion, ginger, mustard, onion, and cinnamon due to which the taste of kimchi varies greatly. Basic ingredients used in preparing kimchi are salt, dropwort, crown daisy, roasted sesame, and so on. To give kimchi more flavor, fermented fish (*jeotgal*) is basically used, but in some areas, they are not used at all due to their emphasis on clean taste. The sub-ingredients in preparing kimchi are 10 to 30 types in each region.

The preparation of kimchi varies depending on raw materials and regions, but the principle is similar. The approach involves cutting or grinding the sub-ingredients (pepper, radish, cucumber, and related vegetables) as needed, or cut it into appropriate sizes as in the case of Korean cabbage, and salt is usually applied to the extent of about 10% of the raw material or brine. After brining the main Korean cabbage, washing (within 12 hours) is required to remove excessive salt and the prepared seasoning is mixed. After mixing all the ingredients, the raw kimchi is pressed and piled into a clay jar. The salt content of the finished kimchi is controlled to about 2–3% through adding salt to the seasoning. With the recent emergence of the health risk of salt, the trend of lower salt content is becoming greater in demand. However, it is necessary to consider a possible shorter fermentation period due to a low salt concentration level. Also, if the salt content is too low, it can be hard to control the shelf life and food poisoning bacteria.

5.6.4 Functionality of Kimchi

The functionality of kimchi is divided into the nutritional benefits of kimchi and the function of microbiomes including lactic acid bacteria involved in its fermentation. Because kimchi uses a lot of red pepper powder, the anti-obesity effect caused by capsaicin and vitamin B_{12} that is produced during the fermentation play a positive role in the human metabolic response for better health. Also, dietary fiber in vegetables is also effective in improving bowel health and constipation. Also, anti-cancer and preventative effects of eating kimchi are being investigated. The lactic acid bacteria involved in the fermentation of kimchi has been proven to show anti-tumor effects and have been shown to improve immune functions (Park et al. 2014).

5.6.5 Direction of Development

It is necessary to prove the functionality of kimchi through human studies to be certified internationally. It is also necessary to scientifically prove its role in intestinal health to confirm another key function in gut health. The development of new kimchi-based products should be promoted in preparation for a continued decline in kimchi consumption. In the future, the government should comprehensively consider the expansion of kimchi-related microorganisms into other fermented product industries.

5.7 Fermented Soybean Products

Fermented soybean products are indispensable seasonings in the Korean diet. It mainly uses soybeans and fermentation techniques that are applied to create new flavors and taste. Soybeans used in the fermentation contain a high protein content (40% or less) and high-quality fat (20%) and a significant amount of complex fiber-type carbohydrates that improve intestinal function. It contains isoflavones as a special functional component, which shows health-relevant physiological action.

Although soy protein does not dissolve well in water, fermentation converts the protein into water-soluble substances such as amino acids and peptides through the action of microorganisms and changes it to a unique taste and functionality. To induce this change, beans are steamed, and fungus and bacteria induce the enzymatic dissolution and break down the soybean protein. *Meju* is the substrate that induces microbial growth for the typical digestion of soybean protein and the *meju* is the base for producing soy sauce, soybean paste, and red pepper paste. *Meju* contains various molds like *Aspergillus oryzae*, which can utilize soybeans as a substrate, and they produce various enzymes, and these enzymes act to degrade the protein and fat, and even complex carbohydrates in some cases (Park 2009). In the traditional manufacturing of fermented soybean products, natural fermentation processes are induced to produce *meju* using soybeans. Then, the *meju* is dipped in brine to dissolve soluble compounds, such as amino acids and peptides, together with the decomposition products of fat. Fermented soybean products are largely categorized as soy sauce, soybean paste, red pepper paste, and *chunggukjang*. Although the production is small, *dambukjang, jjigeumjang, jubejang*, and *eoyukjang* and others are commercialized and sold in the market.

5.7.1 History

It is assumed that the fermented soybean products in Korea had entered their dietary life since BC based on recorded history. The preparation of fermented soybean products was the most important subsidiary food in the diet along with staple foods such as boiled rice and barley. After autumn harvest and farming, the preparation of kimchi and fermented soybean products remain big activities in each family. In the old literature, there is a saying that the fermented soybean products are the best of all tastes, and it is difficult to make tasty foods even if there are good side dishes and meats. There is a saying in the Analects that Confucius did not eat food if it did not taste good. The Korean people treated the preparation of fermented soybean products as an event of great family value and selected a good day for the preparation. The *Nongga-Walryungga* (Chung Hak-Yu, 1786–1855) was also designated as an important job for women. Traditionally, folk beliefs also represented some scientific values in this preparation where red pepper and charcoal addition, exposure to the sun, and stretching an exorcistical rope for the soy sauce jar were presented. The historical records of the fermented soybean products were in the *Jeminyosul* (AD 532–549) and *Jeungbosallimgyeongje* (1780) and were published in the third year of King Shinmunin in the Three Kingdoms (AD 683) in which soy sauce and *jang* (fermented soybean products) were mentioned as items of the queen's gifts. According to this record, *jang* and *meju* became common during the Three Kingdoms and Wangseo referred to the soy source of Balhae. During the Goryeo Dynasty, the fermented soybean products of the Three Kingdoms were handed down and records of these products were published in various literatures. *Meju*, soy sauce, and soybean paste appeared at this time. Later in the Choseon Dynasty, various fermented soybean products were developed. In the Dongeuibogam, the fermented fish products, *dujang* and *hae* (醢), were recorded, and expanded beyond the scope of use as spices to medicine.

In the early Choseon Dynasty, various terms for the fermented soybean products had appeared. These were *jiryung, cheongjang, gunjang,* and *danjiryung* along with *jeupdihi, wajang, yukjang,* and *sodujang,* and some of the manufacturing methods were also recorded.

Since then, the Japanese have produced the fermented soybean products commercially, but the Korean War enabled the commercial mass production of these products due to the rapid increase in its demands for the supply of military foods. Based on this, many manufacturing plants had been built and since have been stagnant for some time, but the production of these products has continued at a smaller scale. In recent years, the production of the fermented soybean products in the home has become difficult and factory-made products occupy the dining table of consumers.

5.7.2 Industry of Fermented Soybean Products

The industry of fermented soybean products is like that of kimchi. The production has reached around one trillion won and their exports amount to about $40 million in 2016. In terms of production, soy sauce is 45% of the total fermented product exports, followed by red pepper paste. The overall production shows a slight increase, but there is no significant change from the output of one trillion won in sales, and the import reached 14,000 tons in 2016. Imports are mostly from China, and exports of these products are to the United States (29.8%), China (18.8%), Japan (6.5%), and Russia (5.3%). As the characteristics of Korean food depend on use of fermented soybean products, the export of these products can be expected to increase as K-food enters the global market, but it requires considerable effort to advance value-added benefits with health as the primary focus.

5.7.3 Methods of Producing Fermented Soybean Products

The methods of preparing soy sauce, soybean paste, red pepper paste, and *chunggukjang* are different than the methods of traditional manufacturing that are typical of those of modern food enterprises. Traditionally, soy sauce, soybean paste, and red pepper paste are used to prepare *meju*, and *chunggukjang* uses directly steamed soybeans without the *meju*. Traditional soy sauce is made by soaking *meju* in brine to leach out water-soluble substances from the *meju*. It takes 3–6 months to mature, and after completing its leaching, the solid matter separates from the liquid and then is minced. This process will turn into soybean paste. After boiling the separated liquid, it is used as soy sauce after storing it in a proper jar for maturing it for some time. The first one made is called *hatjang* and the old soy sauce is called *mugeunjang*. Soybean paste is prepared by adding *meju* powder and steamed grains to the solid matter and it is finished through a maturing period. This process usually takes 3–6 months. Red pepper paste uses specially made *gochujang meju*. This *meju* is usually mixed in 6:4 of soybean and rice and fermented for 2–3 months. Then, this *meju* is processed by grinding it into powder and blending it with red pepper powder and *sikhye* (malt syrup) soup to make it a red pepper paste, *gochujang*, through a fermentation process. The sweetness from rice and other grains, the taste from fermented soybeans extracted from *meju*, and the spicy taste of red pepper powder results in a unique fermented flavor condiment. This kind of spicy condiment has not been found in other parts of the world. *Chunggukjang* is made in the simplest way. In the process, boiled soybeans are left at a high temperature (40–42°C), and then fermentation occurs between 1 and 2 days and the viscous substance is produced to give off a unique flavor. The factory-made fermented soybean products are made using superior bacteria to induce fermentation instead of adapting natural fermentation in which soy sauce and soybean paste are separately produced by controlling temperature and humidity.

5.7.4 Functionality of Fermented Soybean Products

Although soybeans themselves are known to be highly functional, various functional substances are subsequently produced during the fermentation process by microorganisms for enhancing physiological activities. In particular, the functionality can be improved by dissolving peptides and amino acids, which are the decomposition products of soybeans, and isoflavone, which is a functional compound of soybean, is converted into aglycone. The major functionalities have been identified in the products such as in soy sauce, soybean paste, red pepper paste, and *chunggukjang*, where inhibitory substances are identified, and the functions were observed to affect proliferating gastric cancer cells by inhibiting it. These functions are found to be related to a peptide, which is a decomposition product of soybeans. The effects of improving the lipid in the blood and dissolving the thrombosis by fermented soybean products have also been confirmed. In tests using obese mice as models, the subjects taking red pepper paste showed significant decreases in blood triglycerides and bad cholesterol (Lim et al. 2015) and the effect of thrombolysis was also demonstrated in response to *chunggukjang* (Back et al. 2011). The antioxidant effects of fermented soybean products are widely known, and the anti-obesity effects of red pepper paste are also well known.

In addition, the growth of *Helicobacter pylori*, which causes gastric ulcers, is inhibited in response to soybean paste. Furthermore, it was confirmed that improvements in the immune system were observed in response to fermented soybean products.

5.7.5 Direction of Development

Fermented soybean products play an important role in promoting Korea as a representative country known for traditional fermented foods. It is hoped that the government will find ways to strengthen the national status by expanding exports of fermented soybean products and turn it into an opportunity to enhance the fermentation industry based on the fermentation technology of these fermented soybean products. Also, various new products should be developed using these fermented soybean products to improve the decreasing consumption by highlighting the health benefits. To achieve this, it is necessary to conduct clinical studies to expand the value of spices that people around the world are interested in, such as red pepper paste, based on which functionality can be evaluated. There needs to be an emphasis on the role of the red pepper paste sauce combined with soy fermentation for reducing the ever-increasing problem of obesity.

5.8 Fermented Fish Products

Fermented fish products are the most representative processed output among the processed marine products. It occupies an important portion among fermented foods in Korea and is an essential ingredient for preparing kimchi. Fish are treated immediately by adding salt after the catch to prevent negative changes such as decomposition, which is the best way to delay the putrefaction. Recently, there has been negative public opinion about excessive salt intake, which has led to the decline in the preference for fermented fish products, but there is a possibility that the content of salt can be controlled using spices, and other preservatives. It is disappointing that fermented salted fish and fermented internal organ products that can provide high gamma aminobutyric acid (GABA), a neurotransmitter that lowers blood pressure, have negative responses. These can be designed into a positive benefit to consumers, depending on how they are processed using low salt content and using other healthy, preferred preservatives.

5.8.1 History of Fermented Fish Products

Fermented fish products are not just a typical part of Korean traditional fermented foods, but similar products are produced in Japan, Southeast Asia, Mediterranean countries, and some European countries. According to the literature, the history of fermented fish products dates back thousand of years and the products are produced by a simple fermentation method by just adding salt and leaving it at natural conditions. Also, the literature shows that soy sauce is added to crabs for preparing soy sauce marinated crabs, and grain added *sikhae* is used to completely decompose fish to produce fish sauce. The history of the fermented fish products in Korea was recorded in the third year of the Silla Dynasty (683), under King Shinmun, but the history of products used for food was estimated to be around the 1st–3rd century AD. There were salted meat (醢) and salted fish (鮓) in Silla or the Unified Silla Period. Thus, it is believed that these products were already used in the dietary life of ordinary people. Fish sauce also appeared in the Chinese literature, Jeminyosul. The fermented fish products were also recorded in the Goryeojeongsa and Uiseo. Later in the Choseon Dynasty, not only in the official literature but also records of the civilian diary format (Miam diary) mentioned fermented fish products.

5.8.2 Industry of Fermented Fish Products

Among the four major fermented products in Korea, the production of all fermented fish products (salted fish products) reached 44,338 tons in 2016, in which fermented anchovy products (12,864 tons) and fermented shrimp products (76,634 tons) covered a large portion. The specialty product of fermented Alaska Pollack roe, *myungranjeot*, was produced to the level of 2,390 tons. The total sales in Korea reached 321.2 billion won in 2016 where spice products and liquid fermented fish products covered a large portion. Exports reached $11.75 million in 2016, but they have tended to decline every year since.

5.8.3 Methods of Producing Fermented Fish Products

The method of producing fermented fish products is relatively simple. The production characteristic of Korean fermented fish products is by inducing fermentation by adding salt to about 10–20% compared to the weight of fish used as raw materials. The fermented oysters, *gulgeot*, and Alaska pollack roe, *myungranjeot*, products are fermented by adding salt of about 10% and these are distributed as a refrigerated state because it cannot be stored at room temperature for a long time due to their low salt content. Most fermented fish products, which are distributed at room temperature, contain salt of about 20% more or less, and attempts are being made to sterilize the final product while reducing the salt content in recent years. Low salt trends are gaining interest, but food safety problems are higher. For this reason, low-temperature distribution is recommended for low-salt products.

The typical manufacturing method of fermented fish products in Korea is to add about 20% salt to the whole fish, press it into a container, and then cover the top with a thickness of 2–3 cm of salt and seal it up to induce fermentation. In general, the fermented fish products or seasoned products that maintain their tissues are fermented for 2–3 months. For producing liquid-type fermented fish products, the fermentation is performed for 6–12 months at room temperature. Then, the liquid portion of the products is separated and boiled to keep the quality for a longer time.

5.8.4 Functionality of Fermented Fish Products

There are not many studies on the functionality of highly salted fermented fish products. The fermented fish products have the same nutritional content as the tissue of fresh fish meat and are characterized by high levels of free amino acids as they decompose. Comparing fermented fish products with soy sauce, the pH of the liquid fermented fish products averaged 6.0, the soy sauce reached 4.9 to 4.9, and the salinity of the fermented fish products tended to be higher than the soy sauce.

5.8.5 Direction of Development

The results of the study on fermented fish products are not as numerous as other fermented foods and further studies should be conducted on the composition of the involved microorganisms and enzymes. It is necessary to consider the pathogen safety management because there are many small manufacturers that need this support to be successful. Since most manufacturing processes are open-air styles, there is a high possibility of contamination. Also, research on low-salt products should be carried out actively to overcome the general negative impact of high-salt foods avoided by consumers.

5.9 Vinegar

Vinegar has a unique flavor that represents sour taste. After completing alcoholic fermentation, vinegar is produced by acetic acid fermentation by various acetic acid bacteria and becomes a liquid spice-like condiment with a sour taste. The vinegar consumed usually has a refreshing sour taste that enhances eating quality or appetite. Traditionally, *makgeolli* (rice wine) was used to induce natural acetic acid fermentation for preparing vinegar, but most of the products are now mass-produced commercially using superior acetic acid bacteria.

5.9.1 History of Vinegar

In the West, vinegar was used around 5000 BC. In those days, fruit wine, such as wine and apple wine, was more popular than grains for vinegar fermentation. The vinegar made from fermented date palm in Babylon is the first fruit vinegar and used for condiments and improving food storage, or for medicinal purposes. The world-famous balsamic vinegar was produced by the Romans 2,000 years ago and was further developed in Italy in the 17th century. Even now, the balsamic vinegar in remote parts like Montana in the USA is known as a luxury product. In the East, vinegar was used 3,000 years ago. Unlike in the West, Eastern countries used grains as a raw material for liquor. A representative agricultural book, *Jeminyosul*, also has various records of vinegar, including different-colored vinegar such as red, brown, and black. Although the first use of vinegar in Korea was not recorded, it is assumed that it was accompanied by alcoholic liquor. It is said that vinegar is a bitter drink in the *Jibongyuseol*, and that in the *Dokyeong* of *Goryeo*, cherry blossoms were used like vinegar. In the *Haedongyoksa*, there is a record of vinegar being used for cooking.

Vinegar has been used for medicinal purposes with seasoning. In the *Hyangyak-gugeubbang*, vinegar was used as a remedy for boils and paralysis. In the Choseon Dynasty, there was a record of vinegar made of barley, and the *Donguibogam* said that vinegar controls all the blood loss, heart pain, and throat pain. In addition, various records and manufacturing methods of vinegar are presented in many ancient documents such as the *Gyugonsiuibang* and *Sallimkyongje*. From ancient Assyria to Egypt, there are many examples of domestic and foreign use of vinegar for medicinal purposes.

5.9.2 *Status of the Industry of Vinegar*

Vinegar is divided into fermented vinegars (grain, fruit, and alcohol), synthetic vinegars, and other vinegars according to raw materials or manufacturing methods. The domestic Korean vinegar market is not big, but consumption is increasing little by little because it has been considered good for health in recent years. As of 2016, the production of the fermented alcohol vinegars is the highest (87,714 tons), followed by the fermented fruit vinegars (24,732 tons), and the fermented grain vinegars (16,509 tons). Exports are $617,846 for fermented fruit vinegars and $318,963 for fermented grain vinegars. Vinegar still does not take up much of its industrial market potential. Exports were high until 2015, but they are showing a turnaround in 2016. The export target countries are Japan (64.7%), China (12.9%), and the United States (7.2%). In recent years, vinegar diluted with water or soda as a concept of spices has been used as a healthy drinking vinegar and is expanding in response to changes in the perception of consumers that vinegar is good for health.

In the industrialization process of vinegar, the early-produced vinegar before the 1970s was the period of using glacial acetic acid (synthetic vinegars), and the period of the 1980s changed to fermented vinegar using alcohol. In the 1990s, naturally fermented vinegars using 100% nectar became a popular product due to the trend of health-influenced dietary habits. In the 2000s, drinking vinegar became trendy and the functionality of vinegar in health was highlighted.

5.9.3 Method of Producing Vinegar

Vinegar type varies slightly depending on the raw material used in its process. As grain is used, starch is saccharified for alcoholic fermentation, and then it is transformed to vinegar by fermentation. When fruit is used, alcoholic fermentation is processed by yeast, and vinegar fermentation is immediately processed after the initial alcohol fermentation by acetic acid bacteria.

The process of vinegar fermentation is relatively simple. Alcohol fermentation happens when induced by yeast after the saccharification of the starch in the grain. Then, vinegar fermentation is processed by adding seed-vinegar as an inoculant, which contains acetic acid bacteria. Fruits develop vinegar right after the alcoholic fermentation without the saccharification process, and the traditional fermentation method takes place in one container. Vinegar acetic acid bacteria require an absolute amount of oxygen for the fermentation, so ventilation or surface cultivation is essential.

In commercial production, the time of fermentation is shortened using superior acetobacter as a seed inoculant and by aerating a lot into the incubation tank. In general, the source of nutrients needed for the proliferation of acetic acid bacteria is applied to a separately prepared alcoholic solution. It is economically beneficial to ferment in a tank at once and in a short time.

The usual method of making vinegar is a still method that has been used at home for a long time to produce vinegar where the liquor is poured into a wide-mouthed container and left at a moderate temperature, and it naturally processes acetic acid fermentation over a long period of time. This method can produce high-quality products, but it is less economical. A method to promote fermentation by expanding the surface area is sometimes used in producing grape vinegar. In commercial production, an aerated culture or submerged culture method is used to produce large quantities in a short period of time in which the culture is carried out by forcing air and using a starter culture. This method has lower quality than the other methods, but higher price competitiveness. Then, the nonsoluble substances are precipitated and removed from the vinegar produced by this method through an aging process and that improves rough flavor to make it more smooth for use.

5.9.4 *Functionality of Vinegar*

Various functions of vinegar have long been so well known that they have been used for medicinal purposes for a long time across cultures. In terms of functionality of vinegar, it is reported that it is effective in reducing weight, as well as reducing blood and cholesterol levels and eliminating liver fat. It is said that the effect was better with naturally fermented vinegars than on alcohol vinegars. In addition, it was noted that the fermented vinegars with garlic, chaff extracts, lacquer, and Korean black raspberry decreased triglycerides and blood cholesterol. It is reported that the obesity control in response to vinegar has been proven and is also related to improving osteoporosis. It is also suggested to help recovery from fatigue, relieving stress, and decreasing blood pressure. There is a direct link between vinegar intake and satiety. Also, benefits for blood pressure reduction have been noted.

5.9.5 *Direction of Development*

In the future, vinegar should continue to be studied as a healthy functional beverage, which is already known, and the development of seed microorganisms that is optimal for vinegar fermentation should be investigated. This requires the selection of the best vinegar bacteria for the fermentation methods. There needs to be studies to confirm its potential as an inner beauty material with a growing market in the future and pay attention to global luxury products by making products more advanced and differentiated. To achieve this, a convergence and collaborative study between university, research institute, and industry should be conducted.

5.10 Health Functionality of Fermented Foods

Fermented foods are represented by a biological process of changing food ingredients by microorganisms recruiting their own enzymes, or enzymes produced by other microorganisms in their co-cultured ecology. In some food matrices, large molecules, such as starch or protein, are transformed into smaller molecules, or new components are made using the organic carbon food matrix that already exists.

That is, not only does it increase the digestive absorption rate by changing high-molecular substances into low-molecular substances, but it also produces new substances with novel flavors or small amounts of vitamins or amino acids.

The health functions in fermented foods are considered at two major levels: At one level, the positive functionality of foods influences positive human physiology by the material produced during its fermentation, and at another level the microorganisms involved in the fermentation show probiotic effects, contributing widely to intestinal health and brain health along the gut-brain axis. The functionality of fermented foods is divided into the following: (1) Lactic acid or antibacterial substances produced by lactic acid bacteria may improve its storage property (such as milk products, kimchi, and others), (2) generation of dietary substances for improving flavor (amino acids, nucleic acids, and others as in fermented fish or soybean products), (3) improvement of nutrient quality (generation of vitamins, peptides, and amino acids), and (4) inhibitory functions of specific diseases (anti-cancer, cholesterol reduction, or anti-obesity and others), and introduction of a favorable biological change in microorganisms in the intestine, leading to wider benefits on overall physiology.

Figure 5.3 illustrates the summary of the functions in fermentation foods (Farhard et al. 2010).

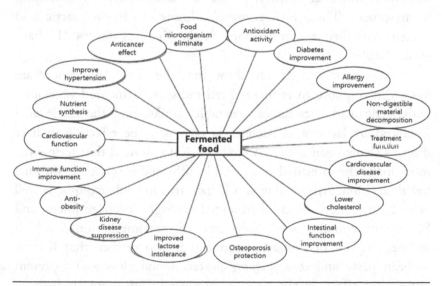

Figure 5.3 Various functions of fermented foods.

As shown in Figure 5.3, there is a wide range of functions for different fermented foods, and the functions presented by different fermented foods are also different. However, not only are there good sides, but they are also sometimes contaminated with harmful substances or food poisoning microorganisms.

A brief description of the functions of fermented foods known to date is as follows.

5.10.1 Inhibition of Hypertension

Fermented milk products using lactobacillus, *Lactobacillus helveticus*, and yeast, *Saccharomyces cerevisae,* lower the heart retraction pressure of patients with hypertension. In addition, taking a lot of whole grains or complex starch rich in fiber used in such fermentation can lower blood pressure. In other words, ingestion of fermented dairy products or grains with high dietary fiber and peptides can relieve hypertension or blood pressure (He and Wheltom 1999).

5.10.2 Anti-Cancer Effects

The anti-cancer effects of fermented foods have been reported by several researchers. It has been known that it inhibits colon cancer by removing intestinal toxicity. There are also reports of inhibiting breast cancer. These actions are also known to involve lactic acid bacteria enriched for anti-tumor modulating substances (Farhard et al. 2010).

The cases presented here show that the effects on cancer are known in response to fermented red radishes, fermented vegetables with lactic acid bacteria or vegetable drinks, and the lactic acid produced by lactic acid bacteria is proven to be effective in liver diseases (Kobayashi 2005). A study on Kefir showed that fermented foods make the intestinal ecosystem healthy and is related to optimal health and longevity. It has also helped treating tuberculosis as well as had anti-cancer effects. Fermented cabbages, cabbage juices, and Sauerkraut contain sulfur substance (S-metylmethionine), which reduces the risk of stomach tumors. It is also verified that Korean soybean paste and *chunggukjang* protect blood clots and represent anti-cancer effects by the peptides produced from these products.

5.10.3 Improving Blood Lipids and Preventing Blood Clots

When fermented red pepper paste (*gochujang*) was fed to the fat-induced mice, the blood triglyceride (TG), and cholesterol were significantly reduced and the lipid content had a positive effect on lipid metabolism by helping to release the lipid content (Lim et al. 2015). In animal tests that used fermented dairy products, the effect of lowering the cholesterol content in the blood was shown and the effect of lowering serum and LDL-cholesterol was demonstrated even when the fermented whole grain was fed. It showed positive effects in controlling hypertension, diabetes, and obesity (Farhard et al. 2010).

5.10.4 Improvement of Osteoporosis

Japanese *natto* is a product that is fermented by inoculating *Bacillus subtilis* in boiled soybeans. It contains saponin, isoflavone, and fibrinolytic enzymes, which are commonly contained in soybeans. Also, it contains vitamin K_2, dipicolinic acid among other beneficial compounds. In particular, the vitamin K_2 increases 124 times through fermentation, which relieves osteoporosis in older women. Also, the *tempe* produced in Indonesia also has high isoflavone content, which shows functionality and has similar metabolic control functions and chemical structure to estrogens and active as weak estrogens, which helps women improve menopause syndrome.

5.10.5 Effects of Delaying Harmful Microorganisms and Deterioration

Lactic acid bacteria play a major role in making fermented products by using it as a starter when producing many products, such as dairy products, meat and vegetable products, and beverages. These fermented products have primary benefits of extending the post-harvest product storage period and producing new flavor ingredients to enhance the flavor. Lactic acid bacteria involved in fermentation effectively prevent the proliferation of microorganisms that causes food poisoning through decreasing pH by producing lactic acid. Several types of fermented marine products produced in Europe fall into this category, mainly known due to the causative microbes, such as in genus *Pediococcus*, *Lactobacillus*, *Leuconostoc*, *Micrococcus*, and *Staphylococcus*.

Fermented sausages improve flavor and storage by lactic acid bacteria, and like kimchi in Korea effectively inhibits food poisoning bacteria while enhancing taste by fermentation. Storage time can be extended greatly with kimchi rather than raw Korean cabbage.

5.10.6 Prevention of Cardiovascular Diseases

Although many other functions are also known, fermented products using whole grains have a function of inhibiting coronary artery disease and are also related to preventing diabetes along with cardiovascular diseases. This function is due to the increased ingestion of substances with antioxidant functions or vitamin E, which in cardiovascular disease conditions is low. Whole grains are a good source of antioxidants and phytochemicals, and there are reports that red wine is helpful for cardiovascular diseases, but it is recommended to limit intake due to the toxicity of alcohol.

5.10.7 Enhancement of the Synthesis of Nutrients and Physiological Utilization

The probiotics involved in fermented foods can increase the digestibility, usefulness, and quantity of some nutrients in the digestive system. Lactic acid bacteria, which are involved in fermented foods, recruit various enzymes when in the intestines and produce folic acid, niacin, and vitamin B_2 and in many cases during the fermentation of yogurt supply trace elements necessary to the human body (Gu and Li 2016). The probiotics in the intestines secrete enzymes, decomposing proteins and lipids, and increasing physiological utilization. It produces amino acids easily absorbed after degradation from proteins and short chains of fatty acids from lipids. Also, it decomposes carbohydrates into organic acids with small molecules, such as lactic acid, propionic acid, and butyric acid, and which allows easy absorption into the body. These compounds also have positive physiological effects in the human body. Overall, oligosaccharides, fiber, and physiologically active substances in grains and fermented dairy products present their own health-relevant functions. The polymeric materials, such as cellulose, that could not be decomposed in the small intestine, are found to be decomposed by various intestinal microorganisms and then have physiological functions.

5.10.8 Relief of Allergic Reactions

The most characteristic allergic reaction relief is the process for preventing lactose intolerance by transforming lactose in milk. Lactic acid bacteria, which are potentially used as a probiotic, use lactose as a substrate to proliferate and decompose them for nutrition. For those who have diarrhea by drinking milk, consuming fermented lactic acid bacteria–based products such as yogurt will help overcome the problem. In the process of soybean fermentation, several physiologically active substances are produced along with inactivation of protein-digestion inhibiting enzymes, which are known to have thrombotic control functions along with anti-cancer, antibacterial, and antioxidant actions. In addition, there are also reports of anti-allergic functions (KatoviĆová and Kohajdova 2003).

5.10.9 Improvement of Diabetes

According to recent studies, more fiber consumption can counter diabetes. Increasing the whole grain intake increases insulin sensitivity and improves intestinal hormone and insulin response. The results of a study on improving diabetes by consuming whole grains are being published by several researchers. Many such grain food matrices when fermented can be even further enriched for anti-diabetic benefits.

5.10.10 Anti-Obesity Activities

Obesity is caused by several factors, but simply speaking, the amount of food consumed by the human body through intake of calories from highly refined soluble carbohydrates drives the excess intake, which is transformed and accumulated as fat in the body to conserve energy. There is an instinctive need to conserve energy to survive, and this instinct is still working until now even though there is enough food. Recent studies on obesity have shown that it is greatly affected by the microbiota of intestinal microorganisms. It has been found that the composition of intestinal microorganisms differs significantly between obese people and thin people. The treatment of obesity suggests that it is possible to control the obesity by extracting intestinal microorganisms from thin people and transplanting them into the intestines of obese people. Along with changing the microbiota of intestinal microorganisms, a method is proposed to improve its function by increasing the dietary fiber content of foods, delaying absorption of nutrients such as fat, or by promoting its action on intestinal microorganisms.

5.10.11 Improvement of Intestinal Abnormalities

Lactic acid bacteria, along with some other bacteria, which are used as probiotics, are effective in improving abnormalities in the colon, i.e., diarrhea caused by overuse of antibiotics, intestinal inflammation, intestinal ulcers, and so on. In the case of Kefir, microorganisms involved in fermentation of milk and grains produce vitamins and amino acids during its fermentation, which improve intestinal abnormalities. Lactic acid bacteria are also effective in improving constipation by lowering the intestinal pH to increase the movement rate of feces.

5.10.12 Decomposition of Hazardous Substances

Enzymes produced by microorganisms involved in fermented foods act to decompose components that are not beneficial to the human body. Cyanogenic glycoside linamarin, the bitter taste in cassava, is decomposed into non-toxic substances by lactic acid bacteria. In the case of bamboo shoots, lactic acid bacteria also acts to decompose the degradation of anti-nutrients such as phytic acid or the components that produce gas in the intestines. It also transforms trypsin inhibitors that deactivate trypsin involved in protein decomposition. Even in *tempe* fermentation, microbes decompose the stachyose, which produces gas in the intestines and prevents intestinal abnormalities.

5.10.13 Treatment Effects in Other Diseases

An alcoholic beverage with acidic taste, Koumiss, is known for its effectiveness in treating lung diseases such as tuberculosis. A sour alcoholic beverage, Kvass, made from oats and wheat produced in Ukraine, suppresses the occurrence of cancer in the digestive tract.

Douchi produced in China is known for its function to relieve high blood pressure. Vinegar has been widely used as a medicine in Korea since BC.

It has been revealed that gastrointestinal ulcers caused by *Helicobacter pylori* can also be inhibited by taking soybean paste or soybean milk.

As such, positive physiological functions of various fermented foods have been studied, and these functions, along with positive functions by fermentation products, have a positive effect on microorganisms involved in fermentation, through changing intestinal microorganisms involved in fermentation. A wide range of studies on lactic acid bacteria, known as probiotics, will need to be actively investigated in the future. In particular, the role of microorganisms in traditional Korean foods is expected to be validated by clinical studies validating their function for wider use for improving health and longevity.

5.11 Negative Function of Fermented Foods

In addition to the various functions that are beneficial to the human body mentioned previously, fermented foods may also represent negative effects on the human body. In the case of fermentation, where protein-rich ingredients are used, such as soybeans and fish, biogenic amines could be produced that have an adverse effect on the human body. It can lead to allergies, increased blood pressure, headaches, and neurological disorders. As molds are used, certain fungi may produce mycotoxin, a carcinogenic substance. Aflatoxin is known as the causative substance of liver cancer and occurs in soybeans and peanuts. In the fermentation of alcoholic beverages, ethyl carbamate is produced, which can cause health risks, such as carcinogens. In some cases, direct contamination by food poisoning microorganisms can cause problems. *Bacillus cereus*, which is regulated in fermented soybean products, causes abnormal symptoms, such as diarrhea, and is legally restricted to less than 10^4/g of final product. As mentioned previously, the hazards of the fermented foods are already well known for their occurrence and are studied to minimize the generation of toxic substances. In addition, the microorganisms involved in food poisoning can also be managed in the process of pretreatment or fermentation to prevent the occurrence of harmful effects.

5.12 Relationship between Microorganisms Involved in Fermented Foods and Intestinal Health

Recently, many scientists in food and medical sciences have shown that intestinal microorganisms are deeply related to human health, which can improve functions in digestion and immunity, as well as affect genes and change the health-relevant characteristics of humans positively and also benefit animal health (Kim 2018). As many as 10^{12} microorganisms reside in the human digestive system, and these microorganisms have a profound effect on changes in the intestinal ecosystem. It changes polymeric food materials, such as fiber, which when metabolized support beneficial microorganisms from the outside or break down from the small intestine, and synthesizes special beneficial ingredients, such as vitamins and short chain fatty acids, to communicate and support intestinal cells and improve immune functions (Rezac et al. 2018). Most microorganisms present in the intestine are in stable condition, but the ecosystem of microorganisms that survive in the colon can be changed by antibiotics, stress, and disease (Sommer et al. 2017) and can be replenished by fermented foods and their metabolic products. Also, the intestinal microbiotas are known to change depending on the food eaten, and these coexisting bacteria play a major role in the overall health of humans. So far, the general theory is that each person has a different intestinal microbiota influenced by the quality of the diet.

The ingredients that greatly affect intestinal microorganisms are fermentable fibers and polysaccharides, i.e., non-digestible oligosaccharides, which are the source of microbial growth, and these substances promote the activity of intestinal microorganisms and are broken down further into beneficial compounds such as short-chain fatty acids with a positive impact on the health of the host. The inflow of probiotics from outside through food varies the composition of intestinal microorganisms for some time, but it is generally not easy for introduced bacteria to survive for a long time and the local ecology of the intestine affects the extent to which it lasts longer. A good way to affect the intestinal microbiota is to continuously take beneficial microorganisms into the intestine by consuming fermented foods or beverages. Beneficial bacteria in fermented foods enter the intestine, survive in the digestive system, and play a similar positive role to other probiotics. The continued consumption of fermented foods containing these beneficial microorganisms allows microorganisms in food to survive in the intestines in which they are classified as transient microbiomes but by conditioning with fermented foods they can stay longer to bring benefits.

Microorganisms present in fermented foods are divided into two different types. First, in most cases, microorganisms involved in naturally fermented foods exist in raw materials or air, so that they multiply and ferment whenever the conditions are right. Several microorganisms, such as bacteria, yeast, and mold, are related by living in the same ecology of a food system and complex fermentation takes place by multiple bacteria, not by a single bacterium based on successions of bioconversions linked to metabolism. The second is the artificial selection of superior bacteria to induce fermentation around these bacteria. Because it uses a single bacterium, it has a simple effect, unlike natural fermentation caused by multiple microorganisms that are in a community. Natural fermentation takes place in traditional fermented foods such as kimchi, fermented soybean products, and fermented fish products, and microbes in raw materials, soil, and air are naturally attached to raw materials to cause fermentation. Thus, the properties of fermented products differ depending on the season, environmental conditions, and composition of raw materials, and the types of microorganisms vary greatly. When these fermented products are consumed, the microorganisms that affect the intestines are different. The naturally fermented kimchi has the predominant lactic acid bacteria, but other yeast and *Bacillus subtilis* also exist, which can change the function of the microbiota in the intestines. In contrast, in the case of the fermentation with pure-isolated bacteria, the products and microorganisms are relatively simple due to their simple fermentation rather than complex fermentation. Products such as yogurt, cheese, beer, wine, and sausage select applicable superior bacteria and allow fermentation to create uniform quality. In the case of yogurt, fermentation takes place by selecting adaptable bacteria in the intestines. Lactic acid bacteria involved in fermentation, along with the ingredients of milk, enter the intestine and represent a function of protecting the intestines and keeping them healthy. These products are of great interest and especially from areas of the world where many people live longer.

Many studies have been performed on the role of the intestinal tract when the microorganisms involved in fermented foods are ingested and are still ongoing. In particular, probiotics have been discovered in the West where investigations have begun to understand the health function of dairy products consumed widely, especially yogurt, which has been highlighted for its relevance to intestinal functions. On the other hand, in the case of the East, there are not many studies on how microorganisms involved in traditional fermented foods, such as kimchi, fermented soybean products, which Koreans consume a lot, affect intestinal health. Studies show that the number of lactic acid bacteria, *Lactobacillus* and *Leuconostoc,* have increased in feces when kimchi is eaten continuously, proving that the intake of kimchi is affecting the increase of lactic acid bacteria in the intestines (Lee et al. 1996). *Bacillus,* which are involved in the fermentation of soybean products, are also recognized as probiotics. Thus, it is necessary to understand the intestinal health in response to the intake of fermented soybean products.

Although not many studies have been conducted on the well-known diarrhea in travelers, it is assumed that the diarrhea is caused by a breakdown in the balance between microorganisms in the new food of a different ecology then those microorganisms in their intestines that previously existed. Currently, in such situations, people experience better symptoms if they eat fermented foods, such as kimchi and fermented soybean products, which are familiar to Koreans. This is estimated to change the number of microorganisms in the intestines and bring a better balance. As the role of microorganisms living together in the intestinal tract is increasingly important in human health, efforts are being made to improve the intestinal microbiota in a beneficial way. Although it can be improved by artificially ingesting superior bacteria, fermented foods already contain a lot of beneficial bacteria, such as lactic acid bacteria, that can play a positive role in the intestines. Thus, it is possible to improve the intestinal microbiota by continuously eating fermented foods. The health of the intestines determines the overall health of the body, and this has relevance to human health and longevity.

5.13 Fermented Foods in the Context of Healthy 100 Years of Longevity

In Korea, there was a long tradition of honoring the elderly who lived long lives, and when they reach a certain age, the descendants present *cheongryojang* (goosefoot stick) to their parents, or when they reach the age of 80, the king granted the *cheongryojang* to the old man for memory of living long. In recent years, the president of the Republic of Korea has even presented the *cheongryojang* to centenarians at the elderly day celebrations. In contemporary times, it is commonplace to see people live to 100 and people have become accustomed to it. However, these old traditions that have merit and longevity must be positive and must be celebrated to build a healthy society by respecting elders and gaining from their wisdom.

It is very difficult to say clearly whether human life expectancy is set or can be extended according to the given conditions and efforts of each person, but most scholars agree that there are limitations, citing many different factors. This is because the biological species on Earth gradually age over time based on conditions of ecology and their own biology. Since the advent of humanity, the life span has been extended and is still ongoing due to the developments of balanced foods, living environments, and medical care. In the Stone Age, the average life expectancy of human beings was estimated to be around 30 years, but the average age in an advanced country such as the Republic of Korea and others is 70 to 80 years. In theory, reflecting on the exodus from over 3,000 years ago according to the family of Moses, "Moses was a hundred and twenty years old when he died, but his eyes were not blurred and his strength was not diminished" (Deuteronomy 34:7), this sets us an example of longevity. All of us want to have and to maintain the form of a Moses-like body and live without losing our vigor at the end of our lives. Although we can enjoy longevity, quality of living is possible when there is help during illness from families and the community for better overall quality of life. Otherwise, without extended community support and social interactions, living in joy with longevity is not possible. Good healthy food, including good fermented food supporting our microbiota, can be part of this social interaction and community harmony to support longevity.

References

Buettner D (2015). http://time.com/3889789/longevity-eating-habits/Chosun.com, The story (2013.11.05.)

Back HI, Kim SR, Yang JA, Kim MG, Chae SW and Cha YS (2011). Effects of Chungkookjang supplementation on obesity and atherosclerotic indices in overweight/obese subjects: a 12-week, randomized, double-blind, placebo-controlled clinical trial. Journal of Medicinal Food 14:532–537.

Bumedsanpharoke N and Ko S (2021). Packaging technology for home meal replacement: Innovations and future prospective. Food Control 108470.

Choi HS (2004). Kimchi Fermentation and Food Science, pp 15–192. DoseochulpanHyoil

ChosunIlbo (2017). Medical care expenses for over 60 (2017.03.07.)

ChosunIlbo (2017). Today World, Chosunilbo(Press) (2017.02.23.)

ChosunIlbo (2018). Science Policy ChosunIlbo (2018.05.10.)

Collen A (2015). 10% Human. Cho EY trans. pp.19–83. Sikonsa Press.

Farhard M, Kailasapathy K and Tamang JP (2010). Health aspects of fermented foods. In Fermented foods and beverages of the world. pp. 391–415. CRC press

Gu Q and Li P (2016). Prebiotics and Probiotics in Human Nutrition and Health. Biosynthesis of vitamins by probiotic bacteria. Probiotics and prebiotics in human nutrition and health. pp. 135–149. IntechOpen.

He J and Wheltom PK (1999). Effect of dietary fibre and protein intake on blood pressure. A review of epidemiology evidence. Clinical and Experimental Hypertension 21:785–796.

KatoviĆová J and Kohajdova Z (2003). Lactic acid-fermented vegetable juices–palatable and wholesome foods. Chemical Papers 59:143–148.

Kayhanian M, Tchobanoglos G and Brown RC (2007). Biomass conversion processes for energy recovery. Handbook of energy efficiency and renewable energy. Taylor and Francis Group 25.4–25.8.

Kim KC (2018). Genomics, Upcoming of Future Medicine. Meeraeeuhak. pp. 143–160. Med: Gate News

Kobayashi M (2005). Immunological functions of soy sauce: hypoallergenicity and antiallergic activity of soy sauce. Journal of Bioscience and Bioengineering 100:144–151.

Kwon DY, Chung KR, and Yang HJ (2017). The truth origin and Transplantation of Kochu (Red chili). pp. 19–55. Jayooacademy.

Lee KU, Choi UH and Ji GE (1996). Effect of Kimchi intake on the composition of human large intestinal bacteria. Food Science Technology 28(5):981–986.

Lee SK (2015). "Medicine for eternal life" Appear candidate. Science Times (2018.10.08.)

Lim JH, Jung ES, Choi EK, Jeong DY, Jo SW, Jin JH, Lee JM, Park BH and Chae SW (2015). Supplementation with Aspergillus oryzae-fermented kochujang lowers serum cholesterol in subjects with hyperlipidemia. Clinical Nutrition 34:383–387.

Park KY (2009). Science and functionality of fermented soybean. pp. 38–44. Seoul: Korean Jang Cooperative.

Park KY, Jeong JK, Lee YE and Daily III JW (2014). Health benefits of kimchi (Korean fermented vegetables) as a probiotic food. Journal of Medicinal food 17:6–20.

Rezac S, Kok CR, Heermann M and Huekins R (2018). Fermented foods as a dietary source of live organisms. *Frontiers in Microbiology* 1785:1–29.

Sanath KH and Nayak B (2015). Health benefits of fermented foods and beverages health benefits of fermented fish. Ed. Tamang JP. pp. 477. CRC.

Schopf JW and Packer BM (1987). Early Archean (3.3-billion to 3.5-billion-year-old) microfossils from Warrawoona Group. Australian Science 237:70–73.

Shin DH (2019). !00 Year's Life Span. Answer is fermented foods. p. 35. Jau Academy.

Shin DH (2021). Korean fermented foods. p 87. Sikanyun.

Shin DH, Kim YM, Park WS and Kim JH (2016). Ethnic Fermented Foods and Beverages of Korea. Ethnic fermented foods and alcoholic beverages of Asia. pp. 263–308. Springer.

Sommer F, Anherson JM, Bharei R, Races J and Rosenstiel P (2017). The resilience of the intestinal microbiota influences health and disease. Nature Microbiology 15:630–638.

Tamang JR, Thapa N, Tamag B, Rai A and Chettri R (2015). Microorganisms in Fermented Foods and Beverages. pp. 1–110. CRC Press.

Yoo CK, Seo WS, Lee CS, and Kang SM (1998). Purification and characterization of fibrinolytic enzyme excretedbyBacillus subtilis K-54 isolatedfrom Chung Guk Jang. San'oeb misaengmul haghoeji 26:507–514.

6

FOOD ALTERS GENES: UNDERSTANDING NUTRIGENOMICS AND EPIGENETICS

KYONG-CHOL KIM

GangNam Major Clinic, Family Physician, Seoul, Republic of Korea

Contents

DOI: 10.1201/9781003275732-7

6.1 Introduction

Nutrition and genetics are important key factors that have effects on disease. They also these have an interrelationship and affect each other. The consumption of food and its nutritional value are based on each individual's unique genetic variation and study of this field is called nutrigenomics. The study of the effects of food on genetic function and expression, on the other hand, is called epigenetics (Figure 6.1). This chapter aims to provide insights on the inter-relationship between food and genes to provide a glimpse of how the study of food and nutrition will develop in the future.

6.2 What Is Nutrigenomics?

Nutrigenomics is the study of interactions between the genome and nutrition, which includes how specific nutrients affect different people in unique ways based on each individual's genetic traits that determine the absorption, dynamics, and interactions of major nutrients and vitamins in the body, as well as how the nutrients themselves may act as transcription factors that affect the DNA.

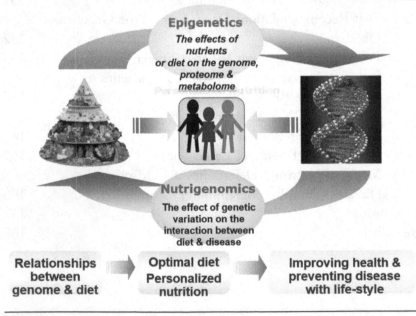

Figure 6.1   The interaction between food and nutrition.

Nutrigenetics emphasizes that each person needs to consume food differently due to the individual differences in food metabolism and interaction, which are determined by their genetic variation. Nutrigenomics is the study of how food and nutrients affect genetic expression. We all know, from experience, that different people have different responses to foods and nutrients. Ginseng is effective for some, whereas it causes fever and fatigue in others. Vitamins do not produce the same effect on everyone either. Some people drink coffee as easily as water but to some others coffee causes rapid heartbeat and insomnia. There are good alcohol drinkers while some people go red in the face and experience nausea after a single pint of beer. All of these depend on the process of metabolism, excretion, and interaction of food and nutrients in the body; this involves many enzymes and proteins that are each affected by genes, and these genes are unique in each person. Oriental medicine describes this based on the concept of "temperaments," and recommend different food and consumption based on one's temperament. Genetics can also be a form of temperament; knowing these genetic causes can minimize side effects caused by certain foods and allow proper consumption of the most suitable foods and with the right balance of nutrients. This is made possible because of the development of nutrigenetics, which makes evaluation and analysis methods easier and reduces costs. The following are major examples of nutrition-related genes.

6.3 Major Nutrition-Related Genes

6.3.1 The MTHFR Gene and Folic Acid

The most well-known gene related to nutritional metabolism is the MTHFR gene. Tetrahydrofolate, also known as folic acid, is reduced to 5,10-MTHF with the help of vitamin B6, and then converted to 5-MTHF with the help of vitamin B2; MTHFR (methylhydrofolate reductase) is the enzyme that is involved in this process. When the MTHFR gene, which has the same name as this enzyme, undergoes a mutation of nucleotide C (cytosine) to T (thymine) on the 677th base, the MTHFR enzyme function decreases. This leads to a homocysteine increase in the body, which increases the risk of chronic diseases such as cardiovascular disease, breast cancer, colorectal cancer, and dementia. MTHFR mutation is closely related to blood homocysteine concentration and is recently being examined in fields like obstetrics for the additional prescription of methyl donor nutrients such as folic acid, vitamin B2, B6, B12, and betaine, if the mutation is found.

6.3.2 FADS Gene and Omega 3

The process of unsaturated fatty acid synthesis in the body occurs in two stages by the rate-limiting enzymes FADS1 (fatty acid desaturase 1) and FADS2, also called Δ5- and Δ6-desaturases. The FADS1 and FADS2 genes that code these enzymes are known as genes that control the concentration of omega-3 fatty acids in the body. If the FADS1 gene has a mutation on the rs174547 base (CC genotype), not only does the body omega-3 and omega-6 fatty acids concentration decrease, but the triglycerides, LDL cholesterol, and blood sugar is high and HDL cholesterol is low [Hellstrand et al. 2014]. Also, the risk of cardiovascular disease was significantly higher than in non-mutated genotypes of the CC genotype of rs174547 (Hellstrand et al. 2014). Pathway Fit, made by Pathway Genomics in the United States, utilizes the marker on this gene to recommend more consumption of omega-3s and other unsaturated fatty acids.

6.3.3 FTO Gene and Obesity

The FTO gene, the most well-known gene related to obesity, is selected as the ultimate obesity-associated gene by the largest number of genome-wide association studies (GWAS) and is also the gene that has been the most researched for genetics-related nutrition guidelines. The AA genotype of rs99390609—a representative marker of the FTO gene—is a genotype that leads to easy weight gain. However, the body fat decreases proportionally when a low-fat diet is followed. On the other hand, the non-mutated TT genotype does not experience significant effects on body fat even with a low-fat diet (Phillips et al. 2012). A 2016 meta-analysis of existing results from 10 similar research investigations showed that diet and life pattern improvements are more effective by −0.18% in TA genotypes and −0.44% in AA genotypes than observed in the TT genotype. In other words, more weight loss effects are actually expected in a carrier who is more prone to obesity. Likewise, different individuals are recommended different diets such as a low-carbohydrate diet, low-fat diet, or a Mediterranean diet, depending on their genetic variation of *ADIPOQ*, *APOA2*, *KCTD10*, *LIPC*, *MMAB*, or *PPARG* genes. Based on these concepts, many investigators have verified the effects of customized diets and appropriate nutrition depending on the genome, and many genomic products are being developed.

6.3.4 VDR Gene and Vitamin D

With the recent increase of blood vitamin D testing recommendations, it has been discovered that Korean females have very low levels of blood vitamin D. The absorption of vitamin D usually occurs in sequences of metabolic processes through the skin, liver, and kidneys with induction from UV rays in sunlight; therefore, people with low levels of blood vitamin D are often considered as not having been exposed to much sunlight. However, why are blood vitamin D levels low in some and high in others even in a group of individuals who equally lack sunlight exposure and spend most of their time indoors? This is due to the variations in the genes that are involved in the process of vitamin D absorption. The representative vitamin D–related gene that is involved is the VDR (Vitamin D Receptor). If the actual VDR gene has a mutation, then blood vitamin D levels are low and there are greater risks of vitamin D-related diseases such as osteoporosis, colorectal cancer, and breast cancer.

VDR is not the only gene related to the metabolism of vitamin D. In the process of vitamin D absorption, the enzymes CYP27A1 and CYP2R1 in the liver engage in the synthesis of 25-OH-D$_3$ and the genes CYP27B1 and CYP24A1 in the kidneys participate in the synthesis of 1α,25-(OH)$_2$D$_3$. Also, the vitamin D is moved to target organs by GC proteins in blood vessels, and the blood vitamin D levels are determined by the variation of these genes, which determines the occurrence of diseases like osteoporosis.

For a long time, many studies have been conducted in the field of nutrigenomics, and numerous studies have been presented on genes related to nutrients and food metabolism. Some genes, like MTHFR, cause critical effects on the related nutrient by a single mutation, whereas other cases as observed in the example of vitamin D, require a simultaneous impact of the variation of multiple genes to explain the differences.

6.4 Diet Recommendations Depending on the Genetics of Obesity

While most people gain weight from eating more and less physical movement, some people claim to easily gain weight just by drinking water and some say they never gain weight regardless of how much they eat. These individual differences are likely due to the different body types, and genetic differences in particular. In fact, from a literature study, about 2,000 obesity-related genes can be found. Among these, the most studied gene in obesity research is the FTO gene, as previously mentioned. Other representative genes include MC4R, PPARG, ADIPOQ, LEP, and BDNF. Among these, the Korean government set the FTO, MC4R, and BDNF genes as major obesity genes, and allowed DTC (direct to customer) examinations where consumers can easily check their own obesity genes without a doctor's prescription. Each individual's obesity genes represent a different function and explains their unique gene-associated metabolic mechanism that leads to obesity. For example, the FTO gene is a gene that helps store excess calories as body fat easily, which allowed survival of stored body fat during times like the Neolithic period when daily food availability and consumption was difficult. MC4R, on the other hand, is a nerve factor located on the hypothalamus, which controls hunger; certain variations of this gene can cause impulsive hunger that cause more food consumption and lead to obesity. BDNF is a gene related to depression and stress, and variations of this gene can cause a mechanism of consuming extra food as a compensation for the stress. In this way, genetics can show that individuals can have different diets to follow depending on the mechanism that leads them to obesity. In a case of variation of the FTO gene, a low-fat diet can lead to an effective diet, and cases of variation of the MC4R gene should follow a high-protein diet to control excess appetite and replace high-caloric foods. For variations of BDNF, a stress-reliever other than late-night snacks or alcohol needs to be found to manage a diet effectively.

Theragen Bio Institute, which the author is a part of, has recently demonstrated a program that takes more obesity-associated genes, other than the three mentioned previously in this chapter and divided these into six mechanism groups (appetite, stress, sugar metabolism, fat metabolism, inflammation, and energy consumption) to calculate the score for each and recommend a suitable diet, nutrient supplements, or drugs based on the score that is linked to a specific gene-related mechanism (Figure 6.2). Previously, there were no standards for people to follow when determining whether a low-fat diet, low-carbohydrate diet, antioxidant diet, high-fat diet, Mediterranean diet, or Danish diet would be most suitable for them. The development of personalized genome testing methods is expected to lead to an effective dieting-based gene-related metabolism.

6.5 Food Alters Genes and What Is Epigenetics?

Nutrigenetics, as previously described, is the selection of food according to the different genetic qualities of each individual to create a customized nutrition. On the contrary, the concept of epigenetics is that food and environment change one's genetics.

DNA is inherited from parents, and it is assumed that that inherited genetics is something that never changes. But do genes never change? Even if gene structure does not change, a gene's function, or expression, is continually affected and changed by the external environment and these changes can even be even passed on to offspring and influence the next generation; the study of these types of genetics that change in life in response to food and environment is called epigenetics. The "epi" in epigenetics comes from the Greek $\varepsilon\pi\iota$, meaning "on" or "over"; this describes the genetic phenomenon where disease and development is affected even when there are no mutations of the gene sequence.

This can be explained using an example across three generations in North America. The composition of polymorphism of obesity genes are similar but the prevalence of diabetes shows a large difference. After the 1970s, the obesity map of the United States has changed drastically, which shows that obesity is more dependent on environmental factors than genetic factors. Studies on identical twins are also good examples for explaining genetics and the environment. Even identical twins, who have inherited the same genetic variation, are often seen getting different diseases when growing up in different

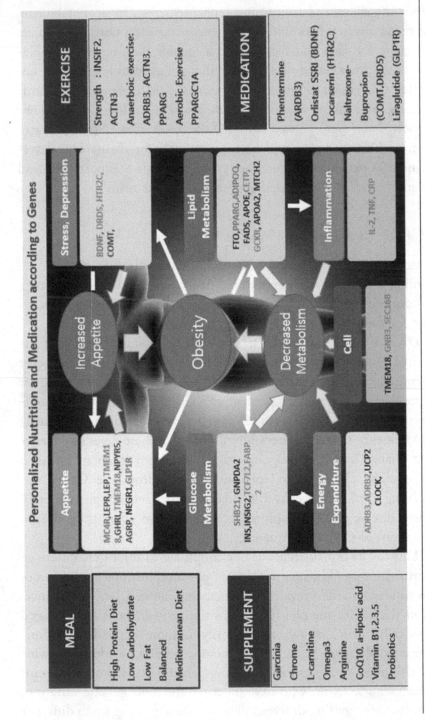

Figure 6.2   An example of a customized prescription based on obesity genetics.

environments and eating different foods. A study that analyzed the genes of identical twins who each had different diseases showed that there were differences in gene expression and methylation, which is an epigenetic mechanism (Czajkowski et al. 2020).

Among female honeybees, there are worker bees and queen bees. While the average life span of worker bees is about 7 weeks, queen bees live up to 1–3 years. Although worker bees are females, they are sterile because their ovaries have degenerated; a queen bee, on the other hand, lays about 2,000 eggs per day and about 2 million eggs during their whole lifetime. What causes this difference? Are worker bees and queen bees genetically different?

In fact, for up to three days after birth, the larvae of a worker bee and queen bee are indistinguishable. But after three days, royal jelly is continuously fed to one larva, which then grows up to become the queen bee. A researcher named Kucharski used a microarray technique to analyze 240 honeybee genes to discover that in the queen bee's genes, the expression of reproduction-associated genes increased and with high DNA methylation, one of the important mechanisms of epigenetics, as a key mechanism (Kucharski et al. 2008). Likewise, birth is important, but so are stages of development. The former is nature of what is inherited, and the latter is nurture of changes in development. Epigenetics is a good explanation of how an individual is continuously being developed.

6.6 Specific Mechanisms That Cause Epigenetics to Control Gene Expression

There are three major phenomena that affect the expression of genes, which are three switches that turn genes on and off. In other words, the innate genetic differences also do show the differences in disease occurrence, but the importance is in turning the "switch" of those genes on or off; major examples of the "switches" include the mechanisms of DNA methylation, histone modification, and microRNA effects (Kim and Cho 2016) (Figure 6.3).

The discussion of the three "switches" that control genes are as follows: The first switch is DNA methylation, which refers to the addition of a methyl group (-CH3) to the fifth carbon of cytosine, one of the nucleotide bases. However, the methyl group does not

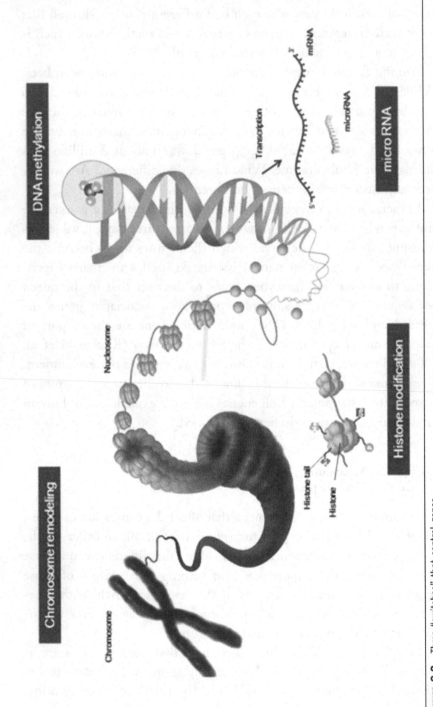

Figure 6.3 Three "switches" that control genes.

Nutrition, Exercise and Epigenetics; Ageing Intervention, Springer 2016.

attach to every cytosine; methylation only occurs when the cytosine (C) is succeeded by a guanine (G) right after it. In about 70% of combinations like this, methylation is normal. The probability of the base combination where a C is immediately followed by a G is only about 1/16, or 3–4%, in the entire DNA. However, there is a specific area on the DNA with a high frequency of the CG combination, called the CpG island; this site is concentrated on the promoter, which is where the gene's switch is located. While most cytosine is methylated, the cytosine on the CpG island barely are and this is to maintain an open chromatin structure that is suitable for the transcriptional factor to bind on the promoter location. As will be observed in detail later, DNA methylation plays an important role in the progression of cancer. The expression of tumor suppressor genes, which repress cancer, is inhibited by DNA methylation; this results in carcinogenesis.

The second switch is histone modification. Most would have heard of histone but not have learned much about its specific functions. The eight histones are commonly known to form a complex called the nucleosome, which functions as the axis of a skein wrapping around the chain of 3 billion bases that constitute the DNA (Appasani 2012). But each of the eight histones have tails, and when minute modifications such as for example acetylation, methylation, and ubiquitination are made on these tails, it affects the expression of genes that pass through and therefore histone modification is also considered an important epigenetic switch. Among these, acetylation is the most representative example of histone modification; if an acetyl group is attached to the promoter, the switch is turned on, and if acetyl is detached, the switch turns off. The enzyme that attaches acetyl is HAT (histone acetylase) and the enzyme that removes the acetyl and turns the switch off is HDAC (histone deacetylase). This is also known to affect the mechanism of longevity.

The third switch is micro-RNA effects (micro-RNA, miRNA). Compared to messenger RNA (mRNA) from which a genetic message through DNA transcription occurs and then carries the message for protein translation in the ribosomes, micro-RNA is irrelevant to protein coding and therefore is also called non-coding RNA. It is also known as small interfering RNA or siRNA, because it is formed of only 18–25 bases. First discovered in roundworm

(*C. elegans*) in 1993, micro-RNA has been continuously researched and now about 28,645 miRNAs have been discovered and registered in the public database. Although the number is small, they explain about 30–40% of the entire gene expression. Andrew Z. Fire and Craig C. Mello were awarded the Nobel Prize in Medicine in 2006 for the first discovery of miRNA interference in gene expression, and since then the number of papers on micro-RNA is increasing exponentially. Among micro-RNA, some are oncogenic miRNA, which interfere with genes and cause cancer; some, on the other hand, are tumor suppressor miRNA that suppress cancer. In this way, micro-RNA affects disease, not only cancer, but also obesity, dementia, and other metabolic disorders by affecting the epigenetic expression of genes related to the diseases.

6.7 Cancer and DNA Methylation

On taking a closer look, DNA methylation is the most researched among the three switches that affect gene expression—and cancer. The dual action of methylation, hypermethylation of the promoter area (or the CpG island), and hypomethylation of the first half of the DNA are explained as the key mechanisms that cause cancer. The methylation of specific tumor suppressor genes that are associated with each type of cancer is important during the stage of cancer progression. As is shown in Figure 6.4, the DNA of a normal cell has methylation occurring largely on the cytosine, but barely has any methylation on the promoter area. However, the opposite phenomenon occurs during the stages of cancer progression; methylation occurs and is concentrated on the promoter area (promoter hypermethylation), and the overall methylation of the entire DNA reduces (global hypomethylation). In other words, promoter hypermethylation switches off the tumor suppressor genes and leads to cancer, and overall hypomethylation of the whole DNA increases instability of the DNA structure and causes cancer.

DNA methylation is often helpful in observing the prognosis of treatment or drug reaction and recurrence. A study by the Seoul National University College of Medicine showed that DNA methylation increases when ulcer-causing *Helicobacter pylori* bacteria are present. However, when antibiotics are used to remove the *H. pylori*

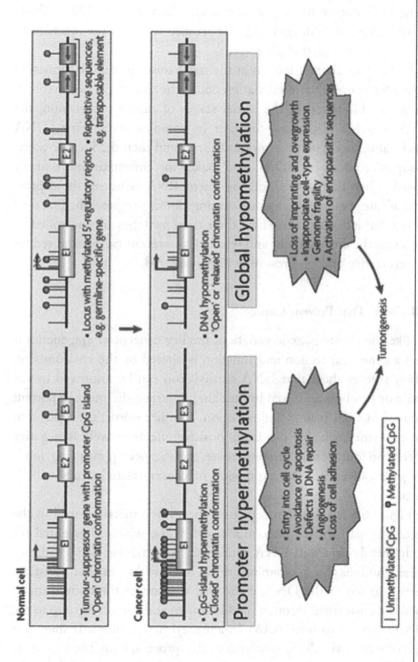

Figure 6.4 DNA methylation and mechanisms of cancer.

Nature Reviews Genetics, Volume 8, 286–298 (2007).

bacteria, DNA methylation is reduced in some cases but in cases where it does not reduce and continues to progress instead, there were more outbreaks of stomach cancer (Keyes et al. 2007). Well-known anti-cancer drugs like 5-FU are also based on the mechanism of acting as a demethylating agent.

So far, this chapter looked at the mechanism of cancer formation with a focus on DNA methylation out of the three switches that turn on genes. However, in the actual stages of cancer progression, the other switches also work together in complex ways. First, DNA methylation occurs on the promoter area, and then the histone acetyl group is removed by HDAC and makes the chromatin more firmly closed. Then the tumor-inducing micro-RNA represses the expression of tumor suppressor genes, causing cancer progression. The next section has a discussion on how these three switches are controlled by food and the environment and what foods prevent cancer and reduce its recurrence and progression will be explored.

6.8 Foods That Prevent Cancer

Unlike the innate genetic variation, the key concept of epigenetics is that a gene's expression and function is altered by the environment. Many studies show that DNA methylation can be improved by exercise or can be aggravated by smoking or stress; the most important factor, however, is food and nutrition. In other words, the foods that we consume each day can bring positive effects as well as negative effects on our genes. Among these, how cancer-preventing foods epigenetically affect the expression of cancer-related genes will be discussed.

Figure 6.5 is a diagram depicting one-carbon metabolism. It is the metabolic pathway of one-carbon, or $-CH_3$, which is essential for body metabolism and DNA synthesis. In particular, folic acid, betaine, choline, and B vitamins are key methyl donors that transfer a methyl group to the DNA. Folic acid that enters the body through food is transformed through methionine to add a methyl group to the DNA cytosine to form SAM (S-adenosyl methionine). If there is a lack of a methyl-related nutrients in this process, body homocysteine levels increase and become a cause of cancer, dementia, and cardiovascular diseases. It is widely known that a diet that does not contain

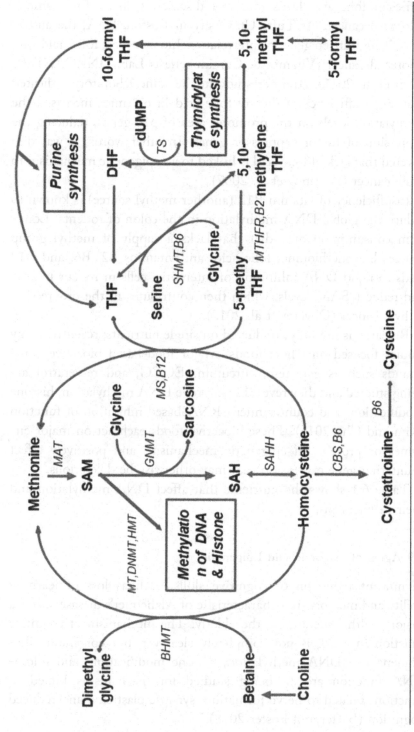

Figure 6.5 One-carbon metabolism and methylation.

sufficient folic acid leads to major diseases, such as, for example, colorectal cancer. At Tufts University in Boston, USA, the author investigated an epigenetic interrelationship between folic acid and colorectal cancer (Vitamin & Carcinogenesis Lab, HNRCA, Tufts (Kim et al. 2011). Another study in the same laboratory indicated that an insufficiency of dietary folic acid in old mice increased the methylation levels on the promoter area of p16 genes, reducing the expression of tumor suppressor genes. In other words, it was discovered that lack of folic acid is linked to an epigenetic mechanism to cause cancer (Pogribny et al. 2007).

Insufficiency of vitamin B12 (another methyl source) is known to reduce the global DNA methylation in the colon of rodents. Long-term consumption of a diet that lacks a supply of methyl group sources like methionine, folic acid, and vitamins B2, B6, and B12 leads to rapid DNA inhibition of interstitial cells in rodent models and reduces SAM levels, which then contributes to the progression of liver cancer (Oliveira et al. 2012).

Research is not only conducted on single nutrients; recently, many studies focused on whole foods. Major food-based bioactive compounds such as genistein, curcumin, EGCG, and resveratrol are being studied and they reversibly improve DNA methylation, histone modification, and counter micro-RNA-based inhibition of function (Kim and Cho 2016). These bioactive foods each act on major enzymes or proteins in epigenetic mechanisms and positively affect countering gene expression that may otherwise be deleterious.

Table 6.1 shows the nutrients that affect DNA methylation and their mechanisms.

6.9 Aging of the Brain and Epigenetics

Significant reduction of cognitive skills, such as loss of learning ability and memory, is a characteristic of Alzheimer's disease and is a major health issue among the elderly. The mechanism of cognitive function in aging is not completely clear yet, but epigenetic phenomena like DNA methylation, histone modification, and micro-RNA function are all being studied for mechanisms linked to functions related to nerve formation, synapse plasticity, and reduced cognition (Barter and Foster 2018).

Table 6.1   Nutrients and DNA methylation

	NUTRIENTS	FUNCTION
B-vitamins	**Folate**	Methyl acceptors and donors in 1-C metabolism
	Vitamin B-12	Coenzyme for MS
	Vitamin B-6	Coenzyme for SHMT, CBS, and cystathionase
	Vitamin B-2	Coenzyme for MTHFR
Dietary methyl donor nutrients	Methionine	Precursor of SAM
	Choline	Homocysteine remethylation by BHMT
	Betaine	Homocysteine remethylation by BHMT
	Serine	Methyl donor to tetrahydrofolate by SHMT
Micronutrients	Retinoic acid	Increases the activity of GNMT
	Zinc	Cofactor for DNA methyltransferase and BHMT
	Selenium	Increases the trans sulfuration pathway
	Iron	Increases the activity of SHMT

Is DNA methylation linked with cognitive impairment is an important question? Several researchers have explored this hypothesis. First, DNA methylation by methyltransferase was shown to affect cognitive impairment. Studies by Oliveira et al. (2012) indicated that the level of two enzymes that are involved in methylation is related to cognitive function. They discovered that reducing the expression of DNA methyltransferase (DNMT3a) is linked to the cause of aging and that increasing DNMT3a2 in an aged mouse is linked to restored hippocampal cognitive function (Penner et al. 2011). In contrast, when DNMT3a is artificially reduced in a young mouse by shRNA knockdown, the knockdown was sufficient to interrupt the mouse's memory formation. Overall, these results suggest that DNMT3a2 is an important component of hippocampus-dependent memory formation. Also, the methylation of activity regulated cytoskeleton (ARC) genes which also support the connection between DNA methylation and cognitive impairment (Penner et al. 2011). It was also proved that transcriptional activation of the ARC gene was lower in aged mice than in young adult mice, and that the ARC genes of an aged rat included abnormal changes in DNA methylation patterns (Waterland and Jirtle 2003). This suggests that sexual changes after acquired transcription suppression may lead to less effective memory storage and cognitive function.

Another example of abnormal DNA methylation that impairs cognitive function disorders is the DNA methylation of the gene that codes the brain-derived neurotrophic factor (BDNF). BDNF is an important gene in learning, memory, and neuroplasticity. According to recent evidence, the abnormal DNA methylation of BDNF in the neurons of mice hippocampus controls the downregulation of BDNF expression, leading to deterioration. Likewise, many epigenetic research findings on brain function and brain cell action are being published (Ma et al. 2009). Numerous studies on DNA methylation as well as micro-RNA effects and histone modification are also being published. Through these insights many studies have been carried out on how food and the environment can improve brain function and prevent dementia.

Major nutrients and foods that are good for brain function are as follows: First, there are the methyl donor nutrients, such as folic acid. Choline is another representative nutrient related to brain function as it is the precursor of betaine, as well as a component of the synthesis of acetylcholine, the main constituent of the brain's neurotransmitters. It is also the main nutritional source of sphingomyelin and phosphatidylcholine, the constituents of nerve cells. Choline supplements were also shown to improve hippocampus-dependent selective damage to long term memory in female Sprague-Dawley mice (Teather and Wurtman 2003). The Framingham offspring study showed that high choline consumption is related to improvement of language memory and visual memory (Poly et al. 2011). Some foods rich in choline include egg yolks, chicken, turkey, shrimp, and beef. Secondly, many studies on vitamin B complexes have also been introduced, which was directed at research on improvements in brain function or increased brain capacity in groups injected with vitamin B complex (Malouf and Evans 2008). Curcumin can be taken as a major example of a brain function enhancer. Curry, commonly consumed in India, is rich in curcumin and is implicated in lower levels of frequency of Alzheimer's and dementia in India (Reddy et al. 2018). Curcumin is observed to act by a different mechanism than from antioxidants, anti-inflammatory agents, and epigenetic modulators. As in Figure 6.6, good nutrients and foods affect epigenetic mechanisms as well as aging, cancer, cognitive function, obesity, and metabolic syndrome.

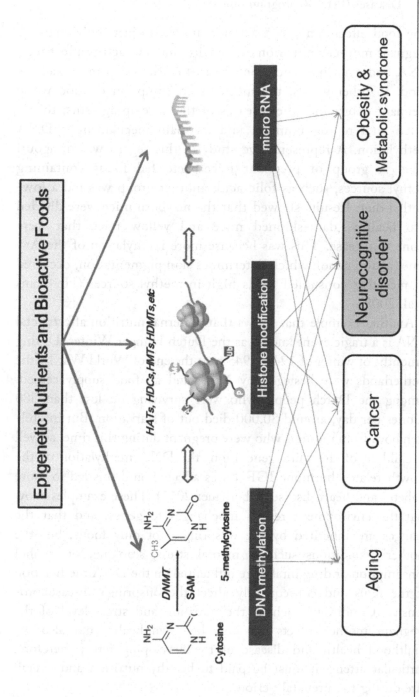

Figure 6.6 The relationship between epigenetic mechanisms and major diseases.

6.10 Maternal Nutrition Determines the Offspring's Diseases (Fetal Reprogramming)

The food effects on DNA are not limited to just individuals. A pregnant mother's nutrition and environmental factors affect fetal DNA and even influence the diseases of the offspring in adulthood. In other words, the mother's consumption of food while pregnant determines the diseases of the developing fetus; this is called fetal reprogramming, and its main mechanism is DNA methylation. A representative study in this regard was in agouti mice. A group of pregnant mice were fed foods containing methyl sources, such as folic acid; another group was fed a low-methyl diet. Results showed that the newborn mice were divided into healthy, dark-skinned mice and yellow mice that were prone to disease. This was because more methylation of the Avy gene (agouti gene), which determines skin pigmentation, occurred in mice that consumed foods high in methyl sources (Heijmans et al. 2008).

Another example that shows that maternal nutrition affects fetal DNA is a tragic event known as the Dutch Hunger Winter. During 6 months of winter of 1944–1945 near the end of World War II, the Netherlands were besieged by Nazis and all food supply ceased. Among the Dutch people who were surviving on less than 580 calories per day, around 30,000 died out of starvation. But in children born from mothers who were pregnant during this time, as well as children of the third generation, the DNA methylation of the growth-related hormone IGF-1 was affected, and this led to more diabetes and heart disease (Oberbauer 2015). These examples show that the environment results in changes to genes, and that the changes are inherited by the offspring. Not only foods, but the mother's conditions such as mental stress, smoking, or alcohol consumption or drug intake are influential on the DNA methylation of the fetus and consequently affect the offspring's disease propensity. Conditions such as the nutrition and stress level of the pregnant mother affects not only her own health, but also the adulthood health and disease of the developing fetus; therefore, particular attention must be paid to healthy nutrition and overall care during the prenatal period.

Conclusion

In conclusion, a person's health and disease depends on both what is inherited from biology and nature (genetics) as well as nurture (epigenetics). Even if one is genetically born with a high susceptibility to a certain disease, its occurrence can be greatly reduced depending on proper food consumption, exercise, and stress reduction. Human gene expression is continuously determined and controlled by the external environment from the fetal period and all the way through the process of aging.

Therefore, epigenetics explains the predictable but important conclusion that healthy life patterns and food consumption keeps one healthy. Hippocrates of Ancient Greece claimed that "We are what we eat. Let food be thy medicine and medicine thy food." The fact that good food is most important for health needs to be emphasized not only to oneself, but especially to patients and the general population for prevention of disease. These concepts are now being explored to understand the longevity in the Korean population in modern times and the importance of the K-diet to overall health and longevity.

References

Appasani K (2012) Part I – Basics of chromatin biology and biochemistry. *Epigenome from Chromatin Biology to Therapeutics*. Cambridge University Press.

Barter J and Foster TC (2018) Aging in the brain: New roles of epigenetics in cognitive decline. *Neuroscientist* 24(5):516–525.

Czajkowski P, Adamska-Patruno E, Bauer W, Fiedorczuk J, Krasowska U, Moroz M, Gorska M and Kretowski A (2020) The impact of *FTO* genetic variants on obesity and Its metabolic consequences is dependent on daily macronutrient intake. *Nutrients* 12(11):3255.

Ellstrand S, Sonestedt E, Ericson U, Gullberg B, Wirfält E, Hedblad B and Orho-Melander M (2012) Intake levels of dietary long-chain PUFAs modify the association between genetic variation in FADS and LDL-C. *Journal Lipid Research* 53(6):1183–1189.

Heijmans BT, Tobi EW, Stein AD, Putter H, Blauw GJ, Susser ES, Slagboom PE and Lumey LH (2008) Persistent epigenetic differences associated with prenatal exposure to famine in humans. *Proceedings of the National Academy of Sciences of the United States of America* 105(44):17046–17049.

Hellstrand S, Ericson U, Gullberg B, Hedblad B, Orho-Melander M and Sonestedt E (2014) Genetic variation in FADS1 has little effect on the association between dietary PUFA intake and cardiovascular disease. *Journal of Nutrition* 144(9):1356–1363.

Keyes MK, Jang H, Mason JB, Liu Z, Crott JW, Smith DE, Friso S and Choi SW (2007) Older age and dietary folate are determinants of genomic and p16-specific DNA methylation in mouse colon. *Journal of Nutrition* 137(7):1713–1717.

Kim KC and Cho SW (2016) *Nutrition, Exercise and Epigenetics; Ageing Intervention Chapter1*. Springer.

Kim KC, Jang HR, Sauer J, Zimmerly EM, Liu Z, Chanson A, Smith A, Friso S and Choi SW (2011) Folate supplementation differently affects uracil content in DNA in the mouse colon and liver. *British Journal of Nutrition* 105(5):688–693.

Kucharski R, Maleszka J, Foret S and Maleszka R (2008) Nutritional control of reproductive status in honeybees via DNA. *Methylation Science*, 28 319(5871):1827–1830.

Ma DK, Jang MH, Guo JU, Kitabatake Y, Chang ML, Anpongkul NP, Flavell RA, Lu B, Ming GL and Song H (2009) Neuronal activity induced Gadd45b promotes epigenetic DNA demethylation and adult neurogenesis. *Science* 323(5917):1074–1077.

Malouf R and Evans JG (2008) Folic acid with or without vitamin B12 for the prevention and treatment of healthy elderly and demented people. *Cochrane Database System Review* 8(4). Cochran database. https://pubmed.ncbi.nlm.nih.gov/18843658/

Oberbauer (2015) Developmental programming: the role of growth hormone. *Journal of Animal Science and Biotechnology* 12 6(1):8.

Oliveira AM, Hemstedt TJ and Bading H (2012) Rescue of aging-associated decline in Dnmt3a2 expression restores cognitive abilities. *Nature Neuroscience* 15(8):1111–1113.

Penner MR, Roth TL, Chawla MK, Hoang LT, Roth ED, Lubin FD, Sweatt JD, Worley PF and Barnes CA (2011) Age-related changes in Arc transcription and DNA methylation within the hippocampus. *Neurobiology of Aging* 32(12):2198–2210.

Phillips CM, Kesse-Guyot E, McManus R, Hercberg S, Lairon D, Planells R and Roche HM (2012) High dietary saturated fat intake accentuates obesity risk associated with the fat mass and obesity-associated gene in adults. *Journal of Nutrition* 142(5):824–831.

Pogribny IP, Ross SA, Wise C, Pogribna M, Jones EA, Tryndyak VP, James SJ, Dragan YP and Poirier LA (2007) Irreversible global DNA hypomethylation as a key step in hepatocarcinogenesis induced by dietary methyl deficiency. *Mutation Research* 29 593(1–2):80–87.

Poly C, Massaro JM, Seshadri S, Wolf PA, Cho E, Krall E, Jacques P and Au R (2011) The relation of dietary choline to cognitive performance and white matter hyperintensity in the Framingham offspring cohort. *The American Journal of Clinical Nutrition* 94(6):1584–1591.

Reddy PH, Manczak M, Yin X, Grady MC, Mitchell A, Tonk S, Kuruva CS, Bhatti JS, Kandimalla R, Vijayan M, Kumar S, Wang R, Pradeepkiran JA, Ogunmokun K, Thamarai K, Quesada K, Boles A and Reddy AP (2018) Protective effects of indian spice Curcumin against amyloid-β in Alzheimer's disease. *Journal of Alzheimer's Disease* 61(3):843–866.

Teather L and Wurtman R (2003) Dietary cytidine (5')-diphosphocholine supplementation protects against development of memory deficits in aging rats. *Neuro-Psychopharmacology & Biological Psychiatry* 27(4):711–717.

Waterland RA and Jirtle RL (2003) Transposable elements: targets for early nutritional effects on epigenetic gene regulation. *Molecular and Cellular Biology* 23(15):5293–5300.

GOOD BLOOD CIRCULATION IS VITAL TO YOUR HEALTH

SOO-WAN CHAE

*Clinical Trial Center for Functional
Foods Chonbuk National University
Hospital*

Contents

DOI: 10.1201/9781003275732-8

7.1 Introduction

The movie *Welcome to Dongmakgol* is set in a utopian Korean village. On encountering such a village, an officer from North Korea, failing to remember that it is wartime, instinctively asks the village head how he managed to lead the village so peacefully. "The secret of my great leadership? Well, making sure food is always in abundance, I guess? Lots of food! Ensuring everyone had enough food at hand!" His response could not have been any simpler. In this health-conscious generation, the list of suggestions to live a long and healthy life seems endless, but is there one you can say that is as simple as "having enough food"?

The focus and strength of this chapter is that the secret to a healthy, long life would be to have "good blood circulation." Is it not too simple, you may ask? If blood flow and circulation in your body is at a normal range so all the cells in your body can absorb enough nutrients, would you really be able to live for a long time? The Dongmakgol village head simply advised to "feed everyone well." However, was it not his good morals and kind heart that kept the village peaceful even when a stranger suddenly appeared? If you look at the ancient Chinese character for "morality (*deok* 德)," its components translate to something along the lines of "even if actions are done in all directions, the heart of all these actions are the same." On the same note, even when ruling a country with many citizens, you can enjoy peace if you are inclusive and do not have people nor provinces being left out. Also, *tteok* is the Korean word for "rice cakes" and is something that is commonly shared with neighbors. The pronunciation of this word is said to have come from the strongly enunciating *deok* (morality). If we apply the idea of *deok* being shared and expressed all around, would it not make sense for good blood circulation throughout our bodies to be the secret to health?

During a former U.S. presidential election, the phrase "It's the economy, stupid," was coined as part of a rather successful presidential campaign. Economy is all about meeting demands at the right place and time. To do so, money needs to flow and flow well! The phrase was simple yet powerful, that it was enough to successfully win the election. This way of how money "circulates (*dol*, in Korean)" in the economy, is the origin of the Korean word for "money" (*don*). Additionally, the story behind the conceptualization of currency being after a man named William Harvey who reflected on the circulation of blood as analogous, leading to the conclusion that our body needs good circulation of blood to be healthy. When asked in a health lecture where, in our body, we would not see warm blood if pricked, the most common responses included dead skin, such as fingernails or hair. A few humorous people answered that it would occur in "a cold-blooded man." On the other hand, from a medical perspective, the answer would be "the cornea of the eye." The cornea has no blood vessels to allow maximum light into our eyes to project images in our retina. It is also nourished by diffusion of nutrients from surrounding cells providing a second reason for it not needing blood vessels. However, the nerve fibers that are spread across the cornea make it impossible to prick with a needle without causing enormous pain obviously. This is due to the fact that there are nearly a 100 trillion body cells all within a third of the thickness of one hair strand from a blood vessel (Figure 7.1). What is more, a needle is much thicker than a strand of hair, so blood vessels can never be avoided.

7.2 Why Does Blood Circulate?

Like in many related concepts in economics, the main point of blood circulation is to deliver nutrients, be absorbed in the digestive system, and supply fresh oxygen, from our lungs to each cell, and in return, to remove waste products produced by these cells such as carbon dioxide and various acids, from our body. As a result, the environment of cells is always constant in terms of nutrients, electrolytes, and acidity

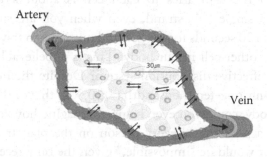

Figure 7.1   Structure artery and vein.

levels to keep the cells in optimal condition. Medically, this response is termed *homeostasis* and good health is what supports this metabolically aligned homeostasis. Without proper nutrition in extreme conditions such as hot deserts or cold mountains, life is rapidly susceptible to diseases or even death. When put in such a situation, the power to maintain homeostasis differs according to your health status. It is like how a warship can be restored when tilted 90 degrees, but a small ferry may turn over from a slight tilt and lead to misfortune. So, how much blood exactly is in our body and how can we make it circulate "well" is important for good health and longevity?

Blood contributes about 8% of our body weight. To put that into perspective, an adult weighing 60 kilograms would have about 5 liters of blood. The average heart beats about 70 times per minute, and each beat produces 70 mL of blood. Thus, about 5 liters of blood is pumped per minute, in total. In systemic circulation, blood pumped from the left ventricle transports oxygenated blood to cells via the aorta, numerous arteries, and capillaries, then is returned to the right atrium via veins. Next, in pulmonary circulation, blood is pumped from the right ventricle to the lungs via the pulmonary artery and is returned to the left atrium in a similar manner. There are two facts being mentioned here: That 5 liters of blood are present in our body, and that 5 liters of blood circulates per minute. For these two facts to add up and make sense, we can conclude that one complete circulation, consisting of both systemic and pulmonary circulation, takes one minute. In other words, it takes one minute for the blood to go from our heart down to the tip of our feet, to the lungs, and back. It would thus take approximately 15 seconds, which is equivalent to one-fourth of a minute, for blood to travel from the heart to the tip of our feet. Since the distance from the capillaries to each cell is about a third of the thickness of a single hair strand, even when you are sitting still, it would not take 20 seconds for oxygen and nutrients to travel from your heart to every other cell in our body. This is unbelievable! Have you seen such an effective distribution system? Despite the human population being only one-ten thousandth (1/10,000) that of the number of cells in our body, could you even begin to imagine how long it would take to send a postcard to every person on the planet? Perhaps the answer to that would be "impossible," given the only recent discovery of an Amazon tribe previously unheard of.

South Korea (Republic of Korea–ROK), as a nation that takes a high interest in the economy, most citizens are focused on the flow of money in the economy. Economic development leaders request those holding a lot of this money, the so-called elite classes, to release this money and allow for more employment opportunities. In a similar train of thought, where, in our body, is blood? Most think it is in our heart or arteries. To find out what is the correct answer, let us look at a typical physiology book used by medical students (Figure 7.2) (Guyton and Hall 2006).

Surprisingly, it is not the heart nor the artery but the veins that are the keys to circulation. About 64% of our blood is in our veins. Just as money should be sourced from places where money is not a problem like among the rich for the economy to work well, blood in our veins need to go around our bodies for good blood circulation. "Vein" as said in the dictionary, is "(noun) one of the circulatory systems of branching vessels or tubes conveying blood from various parts of the body to the heart. Veins prevent blood reflux and appears to be blue at the skin surface." All the key points are described in this definition alone. Now, straighten your arm downward and take a close look. Can you see the blue lines? Next, slowly raise your arm and take a good look at the veins once more. Can you see how the veins disappear

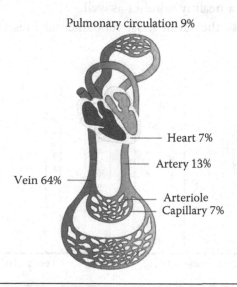

Pulmonary circulation 9%

Heart 7%

Artery 13%

Vein 64%

Arteriole
Capillary 7%

Figure 7.2 Distribution of blood.

as you raise your arm? Unlike arteries, veins are thin vessels and thus swell like balloons when pressure rises and flatten out when pressure drops. They are like reservoirs, which become filled when it rains, and then release water when we need it. At this point, here is another question to think about: How can blood in veins get to the heart? Did you immediately assume blood pressure generated by the heart would be responsible? To find out, let us take another look at the figure from the physiology book (Figure 7.3) (Guyton and Hall 2006).

Normal blood pressure in the aorta and arteries range from 120 mmHg to 80 mmHg. Blood pressure is measured by connecting mercury manometers to an artery and recording the height of mercury first reached. Mercury is 13.6 times denser than water and thus useful in scaling pressure to a manageable range. Systolic pressure of 120 mmHg is measured when the heart contracts, pumping blood into the aorta; while 80 mmHg is the diastolic pressure that is measured when the aortic valve closes as the heart relaxes and blood in the artery flows back into the heart. Now let us look at the venous pressure. It is near 0. It is no wonder that veins are called "calm (*jeong* 정)" blood vessels in Korean. Yes, blood does need to circulate well, but it does not seem to be the pressure from the arteries leaving the heart that makes blood in veins circulate. For total blood including blood enclosed in the veins, to spread across our body, we need a healthy diet and exercise, not to mention a healthy mindset as well.

Let us discuss the seven most fundamental lifestyle habits for a healthy life.

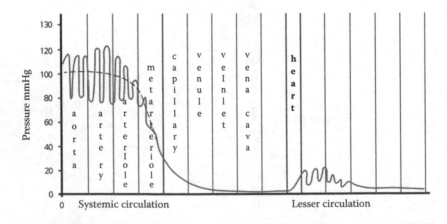

Figure 7.3 Pressure in the veins.

1. Breathing, 2. Exercise, 3. Drinking enough water, 4. Good food, 5. Sunlight, 6. Rest and sleep, and 7. Love, are the seven key habits for a healthy life! Now, we will see how each one of these habits contributes to good circulation of blood and how they provide body cells with enough nutrients.

7.2.1 Breathing: Why Breathing in Air in the Forest Is Better Than Taking Tonic Pills Any Day!

We can live without eating for 40 days, but only last 10 days without water, and only up to 10 minutes without breathing in air. Oxygen, found in air, is essential for cells to produce energy. Perhaps one of the most representative animals with long life spans, a turtle can swim for more than one hour in water without needing to breathe in oxygen. In Korea, people who live long lives are believed to have long breaths. When you breathe in, the diaphragm goes down, and the chest cavity in your body becomes larger, exerting negative pressure, or in other words, creating a vacuum in this space. As the veins in the chest cavity, made of thin films, swell up, the blood contained in the veins flows into the chest cavity. It is like how blood is extracted with a needle and a tube. So, how should you breathe? The answer to that would be to inhale through your nose, and exhale through your mouth. Inhaling through your nose will heat up the cold air from the outside, increase humidity, and filter out dust, allowing for your lungs to be protected. On the other hand, inhaling with your mouth causes the mucous membrane to dry up and allows for dust in the air to directly enter your lungs and increase their harmfulness. One action in which people often do while breathing with their mouths open is snoring, but there is a danger of apnea in doing so. The easy way to stop breathing through your mouth, though a bit unpleasant at first, is to put a disposable bandage on your mouth before going to sleep. Taking a deep breath is also important. When did you last take a deep breath? It would probably be hard to recall unless you have done some high-impact exercise recently, because we do not usually breathe into our lungs when unconsciously breathing. How should I take a deep breath? Start from getting access to clean air. Fill your home with fresh, clean air. Artificial building materials, furniture, cement, drywall, and adhesives all emit many pollutants, and reports suggest that the air outside is much better for the body than purified air supplied through pipes. It is a scientifically supported conclusion that resulted from the analysis of the distribution of bacteria in air. Once fresh air is accessible, inhale until you can no more, pause, and only then exhale slowly until you feel as if your belly would stick to your back. You will start to feel the difference just by putting in a few minutes of effort into doing this in the morning and before bed. This is because this action allows for clear blood to run all over the body. The best place to do it would be the forest. The oxygen concentrations in the forest are substantially higher, fine dust levels are lower, and aromatic substances are continuously being emitted (Li et al. 2009) in the forests, not to mention its green beauty that could make anyone feel comfortable. Deep breaths also help us relax. When anxious, breathing tends to become irregular, and this is where taking in deep breaths would help stabilize our minds. Sometimes holding your breath can also improve your health. The world record for holding one's breath is about 5 minutes, and an average person can only do so for less than a minute. Holding your breath stimulates the respiratory center because the oxygen in the blood decreases, leading to spontaneous contraction of the respiratory muscles. At this point, all cells would be demanding, "Give me oxygen!" causing the peripheral vessels to expand and warm up in response. This is how our body goes through an emergency drill. However, with practice, the duration with which one can hold their breath would increase, and our body's tolerance to hypoxia and other emergencies would increase as well. This can be a foundation to good health and longevity.

7.2.2 Exercise: Why Exercise Is Now a Must, Not a Choice!

Veins have valves that help blood retune and return to the heart (Figure 7.4) (Guyton and Hall 2006).

There are superficial veins sticking out like tendons on your skin, but there are also deep veins inside your muscles. The veins in the muscles are compressed every time the muscles contract, causing blood in the veins to flow into the heart. As mentioned earlier, intravenous pressure is near zero, so only when the muscles contract, do the blood in the veins flow back into the heart. For this reason, legs are said to be a muscle pump or the "second heart." After a long flight

Depths vein(intramuscular)

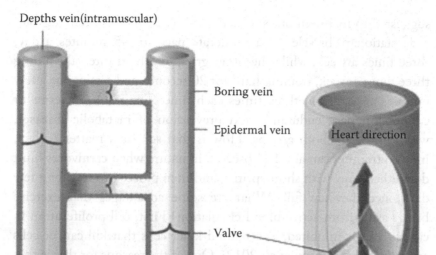

Boring vein

Epidermal vein

Heart direction

Valve

Figure 7.4 Phleboid and valve direction.

in a small chair or standing for a long time, your legs become swollen because your "second heart" was not able to do its job. During exercise, your muscles use up a lot of energy, leading to an increase in your heart rate, cardiac muscle contraction, and blood pressure. Thus, your cardiac output rises to up to 20 L per minute. So, what is the ideal amount of duration and intensity that we should aim for when exercising? Is it necessary to walk 10,000 steps a day? Some may not have enough time to walk 10,000 steps, as it would require about 100 minutes to complete. To come to the key point, the thought of having to walk 10,000 steps daily to be "healthy," began for commercial reasons during 1964 Tokyo Olympics when pedometers were first being sold, despite there being no scientific basis behind it. There are reports that tell us taking a 10-minute walk three times a day is more helpful than walking 10,000 steps in one go. In 2017, interval training showing the same effect in a shorter time period was also introduced. Typically, working out three times a week is suggested to maintain one's athletic ability. In the research, a group rode stationary bicycles at a moderate pace for 45 minutes a day, three times a week; while the other group did brief interval training three times a week, running hard for 20 seconds and resting for a few minutes, repeating it three times each time. The result, in terms of cardiopulmonary endurance and prevention of metabolic diseases, were similar for both groups. How is that so? As a matter of fact, interval training can also be observed in nature when carnivores hunt down their prey with short sprints, and then proceed to rest for a few days once they are full. What are some advantages that exercise brings aside from active blood circulation? First, cell proliferation in cancer cells is inhibited, and natural killer cells that kill cancer cells are activated (Simpson et al. 2012). One of the reasons for this is that the flow of lymphatic fluid, the pathway of white blood cells, has increased by several times. Second, the inflammatory factors decrease (Colbert et al. 2004). An increase in chronic inflammation often leads to chronic diseases, such as high blood pressure, diabetes, obesity, cancer, and dementia, which pose a challenge to modern medical science. Thus, exercise could be said to be very effective in preventing these diseases. Third, exercise increases cognitive ability and prevents depression (Korniloff et al. 2012). Brain-derived neu-rotrophic factors (BDNFs) are secreted during exercise, which in-creases brain cell protection, growth, and synapses. Meanwhile, an average adult aged 35 loses 1% of his muscles every year. A decrease in muscle increases the risk of developing diabetes due to decreased glucose control ability, higher susceptibility to fracture, and decrease in life quality. Exercise is a necessity, not an option. Moving is what makes humans animals and not plants. Researchers say that the house of a long-lived person is predictable in a village. The one that is rather strenuous to walk to and from it. When moving becomes a natural habit, that is when you hold the key to a healthy long life.

7.2.3 Drinking Water: Simply Drinking Water Can Help Prevent Strokes!

How does drinking water help with your blood circulation? A few days ago, I got a call from a friend saying he has low blood pressure and that he feels dizzy, asking if he should go to the emergency room. I told him to drink salty water of some kind if the symptoms were not too severe. He did and soon enough, the symptoms improved. About 60% of an adult's weight is water. Of these, 40% are intracellular and 20 percent extracellular. Water moves freely in and out of a cell, along the osmotic pressure gradient. Our body's blood volume is about 8% of our body weight. When we drink water, it is absorbed and becomes blood, contributing to the blood volume. The increased blood volume in the vessels increases the amount of blood that goes back into the heart, causing the heart to expand a bit. The diligent heart then contracts more strongly, causing blood to circulate more vigorously. So, how is it that drinking water can prevent strokes? When and where do strokes occur? An answer to that could be in the early morning, while sitting on a toilet seat. The loss of moisture through the night due to production of urine, exhaled breaths, and sweat has reduced blood volume, and meanwhile the heart function that had decreased during sleep has not yet recovered entirely. To put it succinctly, cardiac output is not at its best. When you use your muscles, a lot of your blood gathers in muscles, compromising blood flow to your brain vessels. This increases the cerebrovascular blood viscosity, causing blood clots in some areas of defect, leading to arteriosclerosis, which may result in a stroke. When you drink water in the morning, your blood volume increases, and your blood concentration decreases. Here is another exercise to prevent strokes! It is easy. Stretch before you get out of bed. When you stretch, you breathe in deeply and contract body muscles all around your body. Deep breaths draw blood from the veins into the heart, and contraction of the muscles causes blood in your muscles to flow back into the heart. Breathing in fresh air and stretching increases the pressure in the chest cavity, causing much oxygen to dissolve into the blood. Why? It is like when you open a soft drink or a bottled beer, it bubbles up. High pressure causes the gas to dissolve extensively into the liquid. In conclusion, stretching is a very good warm-up for the day as it allows for blood with increased oxygen levels to flow through the body. What kind of water should you drink? In a nutshell, bottled water is your best choice. Have you ever, or seen anyone around you, drink beer all night? What is the first thing a person does the next day when he or she drinks beer, which is almost 95% water? They usually take big gulps of water! This is because there is a lot of water in the body, but even more water loss due to the diuretic effect of alcohol. Green tea and coffee contain caffeine, which can cause diuretic effects as well, while soft drinks can also cause thirst. This is not to say that tea is not good for your body but just that the best way to get hydrated would be to drink bottled water. And when you lose water and salt, as sweat, from your body in the middle of a hot summer day, salty water will do the job.

7.2.4 Good Food: The Secrets for Clean and Healthy Blood; The Importance of Good Food!

Several clinical studies support the importance of healthy blood. In one of these studies, older dementia patients reportedly saw improvements in their daily lives blood plasma (the component of blood that does not contain blood cells) when injected once a week, over the course of four weeks with plasma of healthy young persons. Similarly, connecting the blood vessels of an old mouse and a young mouse by attaching their skin has been reported to stop the aging of the old mouse and appeared to make it "young" again (Castellano et al. 2017). However, continuously receiving blood from young people to stay young is morally wrong, even if theoretically possible. Therefore, scientists are constantly experimenting with specific proteins or stem cells from umbilical cord blood instead, but why not find ways to stay young with food by eating healthy food? The definition of clean and healthy blood is rather vague, but it is clear when narrowed down in terms of blood circulation it is good food. To facilitate blood circulation, the lipid levels, blood glucose, and inflammatory factors that contribute to arteriosclerosis must be low. It is also important to have low blood viscosity so that blood flows with ease. For this, we recommend the following foods.

7.2.4.1 First, recommendation of whole grains, which include brown rice, glutinous rice, whole oats, and whole wheat

The bran of grains holds fiber, vitamins B and E, minerals, and phytochemicals in the embryo, and carbohydrates, some proteins, and vitamin B in the endosperm (Figure 7.5). In a mill, what is left of the embryo and the bran determines the size of the grain, as well as its glycemic index (GI). Refined grains have their embryos and bran removed (Figure 7.6).

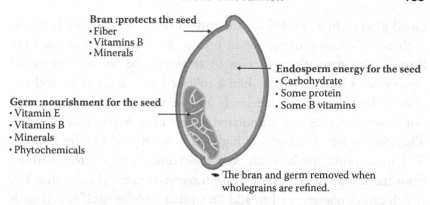

Bran :protects the seed
• Fiber
• Vitamins B
• Minerals

Endosperm energy for the seed
• Carbohydrate
• Some protein
• Some B vitamins

Germ :nourishment for the seed
• Vitamin E
• Vitamins B
• Minerals
• Phytochemicals

The bran and germ removed when wholegrains are refined.

Figure 7.5 Anatomy of grain: The typical structure of whole grains.

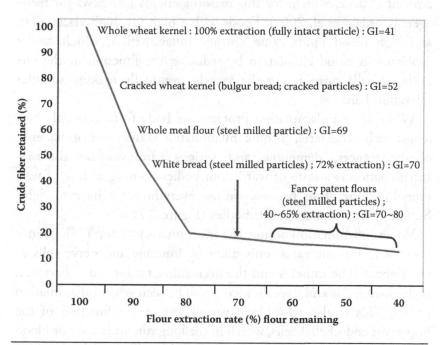

Whole wheat kernel : 100% extraction (fully intact particle) : GI=41

Cracked wheat kernel (bulgur bread; cracked particles) : GI=52

Whole meal flour (steel milled particle) : GI=69

White bread (steel milled particles) ; 72% extraction) : GI=70

Fancy patent flours
(steel milled particles) ;
40~65% extraction) : GI=70~80

Crude fiber retained (%)

Flour extraction rate (%) flour remaining

Figure 7.6 The Impact of glycemic index, cracked particles, and fiber according to milling retained (%).

The GI of whole wheat is 41, ground wheat 52, whole wheat bread 69, white bread 70, and refined wheat bread up to 80. Why is glycemic index important? A high GI is given to foods that would cause a quick rise in blood glucose after meals. This rapidly rising blood glucose stimulates a lot of insulin secretion, and the mass insulin secreted can even result in hypoglycemia, which is the fall in blood glucose to levels below the normal range. What then happens is that our "glucose-using" brain breaks down glycogen in our liver through the sympathetic nerves to raise glucose levels. Our blood glucose level thus fluctuates like a roller coaster, making us feel excited at high blood glucose levels and irritated at low, because our sympathetic nerves are stimulated when in a hypoglycemic state. Therefore, eating food with a high GI make us feel hungry quickly. The main problems here are actions of insulin and catecholamine from the sympathetic nerves. Insulin converts extra glucose into fat, which causes obesity; and to add on to that, insulin itself is a growth hormone, so hence can increase cancer rates. It also increases the amount of acne, which, for this reason alone, is bad news for teenagers (Cordain et al. 2002). Foods with a high GI, high visceral fat, and high blood lipids cause chronic inflammation, which causes problems in blood circulation by reducing the function of the endothelial cells surrounding the vessels, eventually making vascular relaxation hard.

While acute inflammation protects the body from external challenges such as bacteria, chronic inflammation is the cause of diabetes, obesity, cancer, dementia, and various cardiovascular diseases. Inflammation is a state of war in our bodies. During a state of war, everything else stops because we use everything we have to fight. Similar things happen in our bodies (Figure 7.7).

When inflammation occurs, the inflammatory factor TNF (tumor necrosis factor) increases, only allowing immune and nerve cells to use glucose. The muscles and the liver utilize fat instead. Therefore, high blood sugar and hyperlipidemia can be seen when inflammation occurs. This is also why blood vessels reduce the function of the important endothelial cells, which in the long run leads to poor blood circulation. Catecholamine, a hormone that is released when our body is fighting, causes aggressiveness, vascular contraction, and high blood pressure. The more refined grain are the less fiber they contain. Fiber increases the moisture content of the intestinal tract, which helps relieve constipation, which not only contributes to removal of bile acid and other toxins, but also feeds the intestinal microorganisms. In this process, short-chain fatty acids, the main nutrient of intestinal epithelial cells, are produced as by-products. Adding on to this positive chain reaction, intestinal epithelial cells become healthy

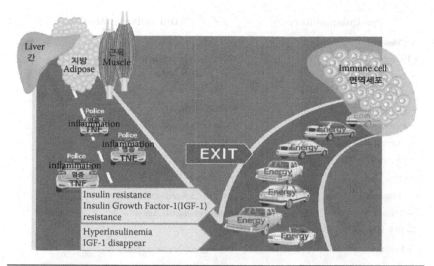

Figure 7.7 Cause of hyperglycemia and hyperlipidemia occur when our body is inflamed. (Modified form Straub 2014). When your body is inflamed, it is a war.

Inhibition of use of glucose by muscle cells and hepatocytes to supply more glucose, mainly used by immune cells that correspond to soldiers. To this end, insulin resistance causes inflammation-inducing factors such as tumor necrosis factor (TNF). Hyperlipidemia occurs due to increased lipolysis for energy supply instead of liver and muscle glucose.

and reduce inflammation by blocking harmful toxins from entering the body. According to a recent report, colorectal cancer has topped the list for prevailing cancer types in Korea, mainly due to animal-based meals and low fiber intake. Fiber also acts as a food for beneficial intestinal microorganisms and increases beneficial bacteria, thus contributing to the reduction of inflammation. What we eat determines whether inflammation is caused or prevented (Figure 7.8) (Garry Egger et al. 2017)!

7.2.4.2 Second, eat seasonal fruits and vegetables Many phytochemicals are found in seasonal fruits and vegetables, which are shown to have anti-inflammatory and anti-oxidizing effects, inhibit platelet aggregation, decrease blood cholesterol, and decrease blood pressure fluctuation effects, and finally, increase cerebral blood flow (Neshatdoust et al. 2016). The increase in cerebral blood flow also results in a memory-enhancing effect. In addition, there is more fiber present in seasonal fruits and vegetables than there is in whole grains, amplifying the important health effects of fiber mentioned earlier.

Pro-inflammatory	Anti-inflammation
A. Lifestyle	
■ **Exercise**	■ **Exercise/physical activity/fitness**
• Too little (inactivity)	
• Too much	
■ **Nutrition**	■ **'Healthy' obesity**
• Alcohol (excessive)	■ **Intensive lifestyle change**
• Excessive energy intake	■ **Nutrition**
• 'Fast food'/western style diet	• Alcohol
• Fat	• Capsaicin
– Saturated	• Cocoa/chocolate(dark)
– Trans fatty acids	• Dairy products(calcium)
– High fat diets	• Eggs
– Higher n-6:n-3ratio	• Energy intake (restricted)
• Fiber(low intake)	• Fish/ fish oils/olive oil
• Fructose	• Fiber (high intake)
• Glucose	• Garlic
– High glucose/glycemic index foods	• Herbs and spices
– Glycemic load	• Lean game meats
– Glycemic status	• Low glycemic index foods
• Meat (domesticated)	• Low n-6:n-3 ratio/mono unsaturated fatty acids
• Salt	• Mediterranean diet
• Sugar-sweetened drinks	• Fruits/vegetables
• Starvation	• Nuts
	• Soy protein
	• Tea/green tea
	• Vinegar
■ **Obesity/weight gain**	■ **Weight loss**
■ **Smoking**	■ **Smoking cessation**
■ **Sleep deprivation**	

Figure 7.8 Lifestyle-related metaflammatory inducers.

Plants have much larger genomes (more genes) than humans because they must settle in one place and survive in unpredictable situations. As a result, plants have adapted to produce a lot of chemicals to restore and maintain their health. Plants and animals have evolved together for a long time so there is mutual dependence between the two. While animals obtain nutrients from plants, plants gain a method of seed transport when animals ingest and defecate their seeds and have helped in the formation of plant communities and ecology. Plants can control the digestion and reproduction of herbivores that eat more than a certain amount, through chemical synthesis and by the signaling of plant organisms nearby (Pollier et al. 2013). If necessary, they can also send signals to animals in higher levels of the food chain to avoid pests. All the chemicals that plants produce are called phytochemicals, which are used in the reproduction of plants, stimulation of the reduced growth of competing plants, the digestion and suppression of predators, and antimicrobial action. Phytochemicals are divided into diverse groups and among these, for example, that include carotenoids and flavonoids. Although the function of phytochemicals is not yet fully known, their importance has increased; they have recently been found to play a major role in determining the phenotype of the gene. When a mother mouse with the gene *Agouti* that causes early death from high blood pressure, diabetes, and obesity has a high intake of vegetables with methyl groups, such as folic acid, it was reported that brown, slim mice were born without genetic variation (Waterland and Jirtle 2003). In a similar concept, Korea's prenatal education can be considered high technology for good health and early child development. Unfortunately, there have been reports that some nutrients and minerals in our vegetables have decreased by less than one-tenth over the past few decades in Korea.

Do you feel any difference in the taste of lettuce compared to when you had it before? It would most probably be less bitter and more tender. This is partly due to a reduction in minerals, nutrients, and fiber, and having been grown in a greenhouse in a short time. In fact, according to the National Health Nutrition Survey conducted in 2016, there was a high shortage of nutrients and minerals in more than 50% in Koreans in ROK, especially in those aged 65 or older.

Because there are a lot of phytochemicals in the peelings of fruits, it is beneficial to eat fruits whole if possible. Flavonoids, the most important components of phytochemicals, are the substances that cause yellow, red, and purple colors in plants. So, you must eat colorful vegetables or fruits to eat different kinds of flavonoids.

7.2.4.3 Third, eat healthy fats There are many people who are against fat intake, but fat intake is essential for maintaining smooth circulation of blood and good health. The main component of our brain is lipids. In particular, essential fatty acids cannot be produced by the body and so must be supplied from one's diet. For humans, "essential fatty acids" are poly unsaturated fatty acids (PUFA$_S$), such as linolenic acid, which is omega-3, and linoleic acid, which is omega-6. Omega-3 fatty acids have anti-inflammatory, antiplatelet and cholesterol lowering effects, while omega-6 has pro-inflammatory and platelet aggregation effect. The ratio of these two fatty acids is especially important. When ancient humans were hunting for meat, this ratio was one to one. However, with the increased levels of meat consumption, the proportion of omega-6 fatty acids is increasing as they are the main source of fat intake in carnivores (Ponnampalam et al. 2006). Currently, for Koreans in ROK, the ratio of omega-3 to omega-6 fatty acids is ridiculously high, at 1:20. Unsaturated fatty acids have one or more C=C double bonds, so they are flexible and are hence liquids at room temperature. Omega-3 fatty acids is abundant in perilla oil, which contains more amounts of omega-3 fatty acids than flaxseed oil, which would be a more conventional choice. Interestingly, Koreans are the only people in the world who eat perilla seeds. Even most Chinese or Japanese do not eat perilla seeds and are not even mentioned in the nutrition textbooks of Western countries. Omega-3 is related to brain function, and so perhaps the reason why Koreans suggested to have higher IQ may be related to perilla consumption. Omega-3 fatty acids are a constituent of brain fat in our body and are converted into eicosapentaenoic acid (EPA) or docosapentaenoic acids (DHA), which are omega-3 fatty acids that are longer in length. These two omega-3 fatty acids are abundant in fish such as anchovies, saury, and mackerel. These are available at reasonable prices in Korea. Tuna also has plenty of omega-3 fatty acids, but they are at high tropic levels in their food chains, so the risk of heavy metals or pollutants is high, and so in the end it could be worse than consuming anchovies. Omega-6 fatty acids are also essential fatty acids and are found in high levels in sesame oil. Omega-6 fatty acids play an important role in protecting our body from germs and other foreign matter, hence preventing acute inflammation. Saturated fatty acids are found in high levels in meat, which are thus hard at room temperature, because they are saturated fatty acids and do not have double bonds. Have you ever seen these lipids harden into a white solid after roasting beef or pork? This is due to the high levels of saturated fatty acids. Meat is also high in cholesterol, which can adversely affect blood vessels and blood circulation. Duck oil is less firm, and fish oil is further less firm. This is because there is a difference in the levels of saturated and unsaturated fatty acids. Fish cannot move when the oil in their bodies hardens in cold seas. To prevent this from happening, the unsaturated fatty acids, which are abundant in the body, act as antifreeze.

7.2.4.4 Fourth, the importance of protein consumption As a protein source meat is important. Everyone should eat it to grow and have good health. To elaborate this further: When do you think people will grow up the fastest? It is during the first year of one's life. You are born with a weight of approximately 3 kilograms, and by the time you are one year old you weigh around 10 kilograms, which is nearly three times the weight you started off with. This is surprising because this happens when our only source of food is breast milk, although only 7% of breast milk is protein. Animals that reach adulthood in two or three years like cows have breast milk composed of 20% protein. Note that brown rice contains about 8% protein. Some scholars even argue that excessive intake of protein may be the cause of many diseases. Animal protein, in particular, has high levels of saturated fatty acids and branched chain amino acids, which can strengthen muscles but also increase insulin-like growth factor 1, which has shown to have increased cancer risk (Key 2011). Soybeans, which has now almost become a synonym for vegetable protein, is native to Korea. Since there are a lot of foods made from fermented soybeans and protein in soybeans have a very high absorption rate during digestion, therefore it is recommended to have soybeans as a reliable source of protein. In fact, in many clinical trials, "*cheonggukjang* (fermented bean paste)" (Back et al. 2011) and "*doenjang* (soybean paste)" (Cha et al. 2012) have been reported to help blood circulation by reducing cholesterol and reducing sympathetic nervous activity (Table 7.1) (Lim 2013).

7.2.5 Sunlight: Why Is the Absolute Mortality Rate Higher in Places with Less Access to Sunlight?

Six of the top 20 medical papers in 2013 concerned vitamin D. External vitamin D administration has been shown to be effective at up to 20 IU, but no more. Unfortunately, more than 90% of Koreans,

Table 7.1 Comparison of autonomic nervous function between Kochujang and placebo group

PARAMETERS	KOCHUJANG GROUP (N=13)			PLACEBO GROUP (N=13)			P-VALUE[2]
	BASELINE	WEEK 12	P-VALUE[1]	BASELINE	WEEK 12	P-VALUE[1]	
Breathing	0.2 ± 0.3	0.0 ± 0.0	0.008**	0.1 ± 0.2	0.2 ± 0.4	0.387	0.027*
Electrocardiogram (ECG)	0.4 ± 0.4	0.3 ± 0.5	0.613	0.4 ± 0.4	0.5 ± 0.5	0.613	0.470
Valsalva	0.3 ± 0.4	0.4 ± 0.4	0.570	0.3 ± 0.4	0.6 ± 0.5	0.022*	0.340
Upright	0.2 ± 0.2	0.1 ± 0.2	0.337	0.0 ± 0.1	0.1 ± 0.2	0.337	0.192
Handgrip	0.0 ± 0.0	0.0 ± 0.0	–	0.0 ± 0.0	0.0 ± 0.0	–	–
Total score	1.1 ± 0.8	0.8 ± 0.7	0.279	0.8 ± 0.6	1.4 ± 1.0	0.073	0.035*

Abnormal = 1, borderline = 0.5, normal = 0.
Values are presented as mean ± SD.
[1]Analyzed by paired t-test.
[2]Independent t-test.
* $p < 0.05$.
** $p < 0.01$.

both men and women, are vitamin D deficient. Expert advice is to be under sunlight for more than 30 minutes between 10 in the morning to 2 in the afternoon, even in the winter. However, this is easier said than done.

According to a paper published in the United Kingdom, the mortality rate increased up to 20% as people went up further north from London (Law and Morris 1998) (Figure 7.9). This may imply the role of vitamin D. The reasons for the role of vitamin D were unknown until very recently. Sunlight has been reported to release substances from the skin, relax blood vessels, and reduce blood pressure (Holliman et al. 2017). The substance known to aid vascular relaxation is nitrogen oxide, and its levels increase with increased consumption of vegetables. In addition to this, sunlight is known to help reduce depression and insomnia (Kent et al. 2009). The internal clock in organisms, called the circadian clock, is set at a 24-hour cycle, and is aligned with the rising and setting of the sun. In the morning, the photosynthesis levels of plants rise even if they are not directly exposed to the sun, and in humans' hormones such as cortisol hit their peak at around 10 in the morning to aid various activities. This perception of sunlight can reach the brain without passing the eyes. Have you ever experienced the back of your hand turning red when you cover a flashlight with your palm? Being under sunlight during the day releases substances that make us feel pleasant and help with our sleep. Depression, on the other hand, is a life-threatening illness, and sleep is essential to our health, as will be explained.

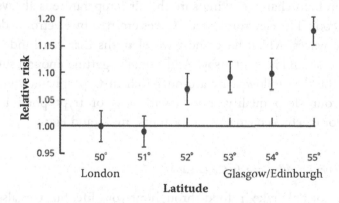

Figure 7.9 All-cause mortality by latitude in the United Kingdom.

7.2.6 Rest and Sleep: A Broken Car Cannot Be Repaired While It Is Running

Just as we cannot fix a broken car while it is running, our body cannot get better when it is up and moving. So, when it needs to improve itself, perhaps by repairing some malfunctioning cells, it chooses to take a rest, or sleep. The Chinese characters for the word "rest 休息" illustrate a man breathing beside a tree. It seems to be that our ancestors also understood that breathing in the forest was necessary to recharge our energy. Women with coronary artery diseases were seen to have a three times greater decrease in blood flow than men when they were under stress (Shah et al. 2014). Have you ever seen an angry man's face? It turns pale. This is because the blood vessels contract. It is the opposite of being in a state of peace, in which blood pressure is stable due to relaxation of blood vessels and a reduced heart rate. According to a report from the American Cancer Institute, sleep is one of the most important parts of physical and mental health. Sleep helps your body stay healthy and well-functioning. It also gives the heart and blood vessels the rest they need, hence lowering blood pressure; and improving learning, memory, and problem-solving skills. Growing children develop cells which regenerate tissues boosting their immune systems when they sleep. Also, according to several studies, adults who sleep five to six hours a day are four times more likely to catch a cold than adults who sleep more than seven hours. This is an indication that sleep also plays an important role in maintaining immunity (Prather et al. 2015). When you sleep, it is important that you ventilate the air in the room beforehand, making sure the air temperature is always kept cold or cool. The electromagnetic waves emitted by electronic devices are blue waves, which have short wavelengths that can hinder your sleep and should be kept away. Additionally, getting enough sunlight during the day, followed by a dinner rich in tryptophan, would enhance your sleep quality. Foods with lots of tryptophan include mushrooms, chicken, mackerel, peanuts, milk, and eggs.

7.2.7 Love: Of All, Love Is the Greatest!

You do not only take in food throughout your life, but you also take in love! In animals, we can see the development of neural fibers and

(a)

Brain nerve cell fiber

(b)

Brain nerve cell synapse

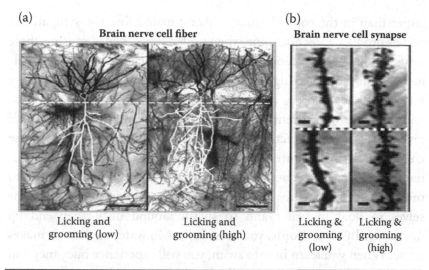

Licking and grooming (low)   Licking and grooming (high)   Licking & grooming (low)   Licking & grooming (high)

Figure 7.10 Differences in brain nerve cells according to licking and grooming.

synapses in brain neurons when parents lick and hug their offspring (Champagne et al. 2008) (Figure 7.10). Likewise, humans are known to be more intelligent when they are being loved.

When beta-amyloid was injected into the memory center in dementia model mice, the symptoms were shown rapidly in mice that were kept alone. When you install a running wheel for the mice to play with, so that the mouse is not too bored in the cage, dementia symptoms occur much more slowly. The same effect occurs as well when several mice are kept together (Lima et al. 2018).

There are cases where cancer is suddenly higher in persons that have recently failed businesses or have other difficulties. Animal testing proved this phenomenon to be closely related with blood vessels. In the test, mice were injected with ovarian cancer cells and divided into two groups. One group acted as a control and was hence left in peace whilst the other group was put under stress for two hours a day, over the course of 21 days. The stressed group had results showing rapid growth and metastasis of cancer cells. The cancer cell mass in this group was also 2.6 times larger than that of the control group (Thaker et al. 2006). This experiment was then repeated but this time being left alone for 21 days was considered as the mode of stress. When this was done, the cancer cells observed grew 1.9 times larger than in the control group. It is estimated that the sympathetic nerves produce catecholamine when under stress, hence causing these results. There is a Chinese character (pronounced "bu 孚") that illustrates an eagle carrying its offspring. How sharp an eagle's claws are but that the eaglet being carried by them feels comfortable as they trust and believe in the parent eagle. This wonderful but dangerous belief gives the Chinese character the meaning "to believe." Another Chinese character (also pronounced "bu 浮") with water in front of the first "bu" mentioned, means "floats." Why is it that water and belief add up to mean "floats"? They say that it is because people do not trust themselves to float in water and so splash around until they end up drowning. In other words, you must believe in water to float. It makes sense. When you learn how to swim, you will experience buoyancy and so will be able to float on water by just lying down. In testament, you may find the sentences many times "Your faith has healed you."

Conclusion

Perhaps the phrase, "the key to a long and healthy life is good blood circulation," was indeed too simple. To elaborate on the phrase, seven lifestyles were introduced: deep breathing, exercising, drinking water, eating good food, getting enough sunlight, resting and sleeping, and finally, showing love. These are also known to reduce chronic inflammation. As mentioned earlier, chronic inflammation is the cause of many diseases such as hypertension, diabetes, obesity, cancer, dementia, and cardiac disease, most of which leads to reduced function of endothelial cells, which play an important role in blood circulation. Therefore, if we provide every cell in our body with all the necessary nutrients and remove waste from them, we will be able to facilitate the unique functions of the cells that make up our bodies. These are some of the secrets of longevity towards 100 years.

References

Back H-I, Kim S-R, Yang J-A, Kim M-G, Chae S-W and Cha Y-S (2011). Effects of Chungkookjang supplementation on obesity and atherosclerotic indices in overweight/obese subjects: A 12-week, randomized, double-blind, placebo-controlled clinical trial. *Journal of Medicinal Food* 14:532–537.

Castellano JM, Mosher KI, Abbey RJ, McBride AA, James ML, Berdnik D, Shen JC, Zou B, Xie XS and Tingle M (2017). Human umbilical cord plasma proteins revitalize hippocampal function in aged mice. *Nature* 544:488–492.

Cha Y-S, Yang J-A, Back H-I, Kim S-R, Kim M-G, Jung S-J, Song WO and Chae S-W (2012). Visceral fat and body weight are reduced in overweight adults by the supplementation of Doenjang, a fermented soybean paste. *Nutrition Research and Practice* 6:520–526.

Champagne DL, Bagot RC, van Hasselt F, Ramakers G, Meaney MJ, De Kloet ER, Joëls M and Krugers H (2008). Maternal care and hippocampal plasticity: evidence for experience-dependent structural plasticity, altered synaptic functioning, and differential responsiveness to glucocorticoids and stress. *Journal of Neuroscience* 28:6037–6045.

Colbert LH, Visser M, Simonsick EM, Tracy RP, Newman AB, Kritchevsky SB, Pahor M, Taaffe DR, Brach J and Rubin S (2004). Physical activity, exercise, and inflammatory markers in older adults: Findings from the Health, Aging and Body Composition Study. *Journal of the American Geriatrics Society* 52:1098–1104.

Cordain L, Lindeberg S, Hurtado M, Hill K, Eaton SB and Brand-Miller J (2002). Acne vulgaris: a disease of Western civilization. *Archives of Dermatology* 138:1584–1590.

Egger G, Binns A, Rossner S and Saner M (2017). *Lifestyle Medicine: Lifestyle, The Environment and Preventive Medicine in Health and Disease.* Academic Press.

Guyton AC and Hall JE (2006). Medical physiology. *Gökhan N, Çavuşoğlu H (Çeviren)* 3:162–163, 78, 162.

Holliman G, Lowe D, Cohen H, Felton S and Raj K (2017). Ultraviolet radiation-induced production of nitric oxide: a multi-cell and multi-donor analysis. *Scientific Reports* 7:1–11.

Kent ST, McClure LA, Crosson WL, Arnett DK, Wadley VG and Sathiakumar N (2009). Effect of sunlight exposure on cognitive function among depressed and non-depressed participants: a REGARDS cross-sectional study. *Environmental Health* 8:1–14.

Key TJ (2011). Diet, insulin-like growth factor-1 and cancer risk. *Proceedings of the Nutrition Society* 70:385–388.

Korniloff, K, Vanhala M, Kautiainen H, Koponen H, Peltonen M, Mäntyselkä P, Oksa H, Kampman O and Häkkinen A (2012). Lifetime leisure-time physical activity and the risk of depressive symptoms at the ages of 65–74 years: the FIN-D2D survey. *Preventive medicine* 54:313–315.

Law M and Morris J (1998). Why is mortality higher in poorer areas and in more northern areas of England and Wales? *Journal of Epidemiology & Community Health* 52:344–352.

Li Q, Kobayashi M, Wakayama Y, Inagaki H, Katsumata M, Hirata Y, Hirata K, Shimizu T, Kawada T and Park B (2009). Effect of phytoncide from trees on human natural killer cell function. *International Journal of Immunopathology and Pharmacology* 22:951–959.

Lim JH (2013). The effect of Kochujang pills on blood lipids profiles in hyperlipidemia subjects: A 12 weeks, randomized, double-blind, placebo-controlled clinical trial. *Chonbuk National University Master* 52:38–52.

Lima MGP, Schimidt HL, Garcia A, Daré LR, Carpes FP, Izquierdo I and Mello-Carpes PB (2018). Environmental enrichment and exercise are better than social enrichment to reduce memory deficits in amyloid beta neurotoxicity. *Proceedings of the National Academy of Sciences* 115:E2403–E2409.

Neshatdoust S, Saunders C, Castle SM, Vauzour D, Williams C, Butler L, Lovegrove JA and Spencer JP (2016). High-flavonoid intake induces cognitive improvements linked to changes in serum brain-derived neurotrophic factor: two randomised, controlled trials. *Nutrition and Healthy Aging* 4:81–93.

Pollier J, Moses T, González-Guzmán M, De Geyter N, Lippens S, Bossche RV, Marhavý P, Kremer A, Morreel K and Guérin CJ (2013). The protein quality control system manages plant defence compound synthesis. *Nature* 504:148–152.

Ponnampalam E, Mann N and Sinclair A (2006). Effect of feeding systems on omega-3 fatty acids, conjugated linoleic acid and trans fatty acids in Australian beef cuts: potential impact on humnan health. *Asia Pacific Journal of Clinical Nutrition* 15:21–29.

Prather AA, Janicki-Deverts D, Hall MH and Cohen S (2015). Behaviorally assessed sleep and susceptibility to the common cold. *Sleep* 38:1353–1359.

Shah AJ, Ghasemzadeh N, Zaragoza-Macias E, Patel R, Eapen DJ, Neeland IJ, Pimple PM, Zafari AM, Quyyumi AA and Vaccarino V (2014). Sex and age differences in the association of depression with obstructive coronary artery disease and adverse cardiovascular events. *Journal of the American Heart Association*, 3:e000741.

Simpson RJ, Lowder TW, Spielmann G, Bigley AB, LaVoy EC and Kunz H (2012). Exercise and the aging immune system. *Ageing Research Reviews* 11:404–420.

Straub RH (2014). Insulin resistance, selfish brain, and selfish immune system: an evolutionarily positively selected program used in chronic inflammatory diseases. *Arthritis Research & Therapy* 16(Suppl 2), S4:1–15.

Thaker PH, Han LY, Kamat AA, Arevalo JM, Takahashi R, Lu C, Jennings NB, Armaiz-Pena G, Bankson JA and Ravoori M (2006). Chronic stress promotes tumor growth and angiogenesis in a mouse model of ovarian carcinoma. *Nature Medicine* 12:939–944.

Waterland RA and Jirtle RL (2003). Transposable elements: targets for early nutritional effects on epigenetic gene regulation. *Molecular and Cellular Biology* 23:5293–5300.

8

HEALTH FUNCTIONAL FOOD MARKET IS THE TREND

HYUN WOO KIM, SEA MI PARK, GYU HAN JO, SUN MIN KIM, AND HYUN JIN PARK

Department of Biotechnology,
College of Life Science and
Biotechnology, Korea University,
Republic of Korea

Contents

8.1 Introduction: The History and Origin of Health-Targeted Functional Foods

With the recent aging of the population, there is a growing interest in health-targeted functionality of foods throughout the global food industry. This is reflected in the increased consciousness and overall awareness of food, which is the basis of life and, as a result, health-targeted functional foods are steadily gaining popularity as interest in personal health care is increasing. Food is no longer responsible for hunger or supplementing nutrients but must also must be able to meet the need for health promotion and wellness.

The concept of health-targeted functionality in food is presumed to have been generalized in the late 1980s when the term *functional*

DOI: 10.1201/9781003275732-9

food was first used in Japan (Weststrate et al. 2002). But beyond what is known, functional food has a long history. In Korea, China, Japan, and other Asian countries, the relationship between numerous kinds of food and certain health benefits has traditionally been introduced and understood as part of living. In modern history, medicine and food are regarded as separate and distinct, but in the past, the idea that food and medicine are fundamentally the same was widely used. The oldest book, *Shin non bon cho gyeong*, introduces 365 kinds of foods into upper, middle, and lower types (Park 2012). First is a common diet to eat for a long time because it is not poisonous; second is food that is used for a long time to protect the body, that is, medicine; and third, food that is used for acute illness and cannot be used for a long time, which is classified as a medicinal food and as a toxic food if taken regularly. From this point of view, we can see that the concept of food and medicine as part of the same integral domain, which has already been established in our daily diet (Figure 8.1).

Korea established the "Nutritional Products" system of the Food Sanitation Act of 1977 on functional foods, and the concept and legal basis for health functional foods began to be established in earnest. Therefore, in 1987, the food group presented the use of health-

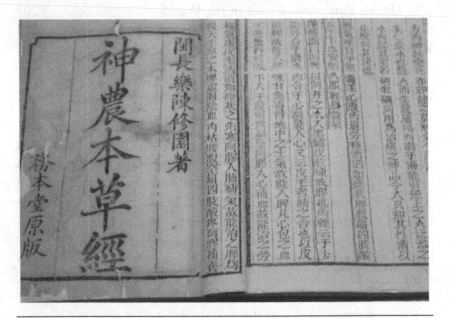

Figure 8.1   *Shin non bon cho gyeong* (China's first professional pharmacy book).

targeted use for infants, patients, and pregnant women. By 1989, 21 health supplemental food systems were created and separated them from special nutrition foods. In addition, in line with international trends, "the Act on Health Functional Foods (abbreviation: Health Functional Foods Act)" was promulgated for the first time in August 2002, and in 2004, the system and standards on food functionality and safety were established (Figure 8.2). The law aims to contribute to the promotion of health and the protection of consumers by securing the safety and quality of health functional foods and promoting their wholesome distribution and sales (Article 1 of the Health Functional Food Act).

However, the side effects of functional foods, which has flooded the market with a lot of products in a short period of time, are bad. First, it is difficult to properly manage the rapidly expanding functional foods, when it is expanded and aligned to similar food groups that are easy to permit as otherwise it is not easy to enter the market for new materials and new products. As a result, even though it is not a medicine for treating diseases, many negative consumer behaviors and lack of benefits have occurred due to hype and false advertising, and the perception of health-targeted functional foods has been distorted. In addition, many potential side effects are caused by indiscriminate intake and therefore consumers need wisdom to properly consume functional foods for health benefits.

Therefore, this chapter explores definitions for proper understanding of functional foods targeted for health benefits, functions, and efficacy according to classification criteria, and management of

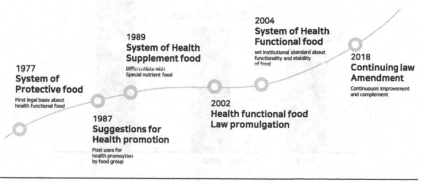

Figure 8.2   Korean laws related to health-targeted functional foods.

health-targeted functional food by country. In addition, this chapter will examine how the development of modern food science and technology can influence functional foods for health benefits in the future. We hope that this will help anyone who is interested in health as well as relevancy of functional foods for health such as scientists and policy makers in the government and organizations.

8.2 The Golden Age of Health Functional Food

The desire of the Republic of Korea (ROK) for healthy and pleasant retirement is increasing, rather than simply living long and this is centered on the elderly population with economic power. In addition, investments for their own health are increasing, especially among young people with purchasing power. As a result, the domestic functional food market is steadily growing, and the types of functional foods and distribution channels are also diversifying. In 2017, the size of the functional food market in Korea was 3.89 trillion won, which was nearly 900 billion won higher compared to 2.99 trillion won in 2015. Not only the market size but also its growth rate has rapidly increased to 10.5% in 2016 and 17.2% in 2017 (Figure 8.3) (Korea Health Supplements Association 2017).

Since the 1980s, when the foundation for functional foods was established, various foods with health-relevant functionality were introduced. It is interesting to note that the health-targeted functional interests of the food industry began with preference foods.

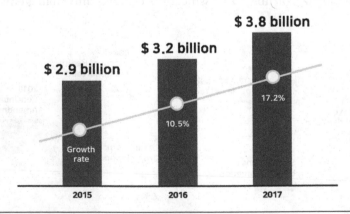

Figure 8.3   Health-targeted functional food domestic market.

Launched in 1985, the product called "No No Gum" is the first functional food that can remove bad breath without using sugar (Kim et al. 2016). Since then, gum, which has been officially recognized as a functional ingredient to help reduce the risk of tooth decay, has been released, accounting for more than 50% of the entire market. Since then, the competition in the beverage market started using functional fiber, taurine, vitamins, etc., and the slogan for drinking based on health has continued to this day. In recent years, all types of foods, such as supplements, rice, and beverages, have been given functionality attributes. It is now the era of health-targeted functional foods.

In the late 2000s, as well-being became a major social issue, health functional foods such as red ginseng became popular. Since 2010, the growing interest in women's and children's health has led to the development of products that relieve women's menopausal symptoms, and products that can help children grow without obstacles. Furthermore, the concept of inner beauty that directly allows ingestion of healthy ingredients that are helpful for overall beauty has become a new trend. As a result, various products that are good for skin and eye health are entering into the market (Figure 8.4). Meanwhile, well-aging products for young and healthy lives are

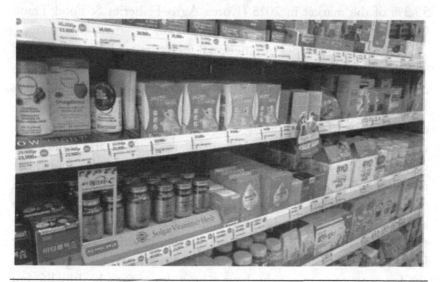

Figure 8.4 Various inner beauty products in market.

expanding, especially for those in their 50s and 60s, and products that can improve menopause and hair loss are mainly sold.

Recently, products related to boosting immunity have been gaining popularity under the influence of the viral infection MERS. In particular, products such as spirulina, probiotics, and red ginseng were mainly introduced to the market. Spirulina is composed of about 70% protein, which is known to help improve immunity. In addition, probiotics not only promote intestinal movement, but also help to improve immunity by balancing intestinal bacteria, and finally, red ginseng contains a large amount of saponin to help boost immunity.

In addition, the health functional food market, which was previously concentrated only on red ginseng, has diversified into probiotics, multivitamin, and EPA- and DHA-containing fats and oils (omega-3). As a result, age groups purchasing functional foods are widening from young children to examinees, young people, middle-aged, and elderly people. As the market grew and the choice of products expanded, so did the distribution channels. For example, the number of purchases through the internet mall, where it is easy to compare the efficacy and price of each functional food product, has been increasing, especially among young people. However, as the elderly population is also increasing, direct sales channels such as door-to-door sales and multi-stage sales for the elderly account for 55.3% of the market in 2015 (Korea Agro-Fisheries & Food Trade Corporation 2016).

As these various types of functional foods are sold through various distribution channels, they are loved by all ages. But there is one drawback to such health functional foods: They are expensive. Recently, private-label (PL) products have been developed to solve this problem. PL refers to its own brand of products made by distributors, which can reduce the cost of trademarks and reduce advertising costs. Initially PL products were mostly general foods, but recently, large distribution companies have developed and marketed functional foods for health such as vitamins, red ginseng, and lutein as PL products. The main attraction of PL functional foods is that they potentially have a similar effect to other branded products but at lower prices. Therefore, it is expected that the market will grow with the focus on consumers who have a high desire for a healthy life but low purchasing power.

8.3 Health Functional Food That Is Good to Know and Understand

Most people want to lead a healthy life by eating food. The function of food can be divided into three areas. The primary function of food is "nutritional function." This means that nutrients in food play a role in sustaining life in the short and long term. The second function is "sense function," which is the function viewed from the sensory and symbolic aspects of food taste, aroma, and physical properties. The third function of food is "bioregulatory function," and various biologically active ingredients in foods help improve health and prevent disease. Health functional foods can be said to be a group of foods focused on bioregulatory function, the third function of food. To prevent disease and maintain a healthy life and therefore the characteristics of dietary supplements that contemporary population frequently consume are discussed.

Not all foods are good for health, but not all of them are health foods. Health-targeted functional foods are often confused with healthy foods and health supplements, but there are clear differences between health-targeted functional foods based on bioregulatory function and other food groups (Table 8.1).

Table 8.1 Difference between health food, health supplement food, and health functional food

	HEALTH FOOD	HEALTH SUPPLEMENT FOOD	HEALTH-TARGETED FUNCTIONAL FOOD
Characteristic	• Commonly referred to as foods that can be expected to improve health • A concept that encompasses foods that help health, such as health supplements	• Foods that have been manufactured and processed by separating certain ingredients in anticipation that certain ingredients of the food will be useful in the body. • Safety and functionality were not recognized by KFDA	• Foods that are manufactured and processed with raw materials or ingredients that are useful for the human body based on bioregulatory function. • Products recognized for safety and health-targeted functionality from the KFDA
Related Law	Not legally defined	Korea food standards codex	Korea health functional food standards codex
Example Product	Deer antler, Chaga mushroom	Royal jelly processed food, enzyme food	Vitamin C, red ginseng extract

Since health foods are not clearly defined by law, the boundaries between general foods and health foods are vague. This is a concept encompassing all foods that are good for health, health supplements, nutritional supplements, etc. are all health foods. Health supplements, which are most likely to be confused with health foods, are described in the Korean Food Standards Codex as "Food prepared and processed by separating, extracting, extracting, enriching, refining, mixing, etc. the ingredients contained in the food source ash for the purpose of ingesting them in anticipation of their usefulness in physical and physiological terms." In other words, health supplements are foods processed by separating only certain components from foods. To date, 24 items have been listed as food supplements in the Korean Food Standards Codex, including refined fish oil processed foods, royal jelly processed foods, and enzyme foods.

According to the Act on Health Functional Foods provided by the Ministry of Food and Drug Safety, health functional foods are foods made from raw materials or ingredients with functional health property or health function (health-targeted) useful to the human body (Article 3 of Law for Health Functional Foods). Only raw materials approved by the Ministry of Food and Drug Safety as functional have been processed for easy consumption such as tablets, capsules, and liquids. In the Korean Food Standards Codex "Functionality" at this time is specified in the health functional foods to obtain useful effects on health use, such as nutrient control or physiological effects on the structure and function of the human body. The difference between dietary supplements and other food groups is that the functionality of the ingredients has been confirmed by health-relevant scientific evidence. It is classified into three types according to what functions are shown in the body label from evaluation of studies on efficacy (Table 8.2) (Ministry of Food and Drug Safety 2016).

The disease risk reduction function is a function that can reduce the incidence of disease or deterioration of health when eating food. This is only admitted if there is sufficient scientific evidence on functionality to help reduce the incidence of disease. Only a high level of evidence of functionality is recognized as a function of reducing disease risk, so the raw materials are limited.

Table 8.2 Characteristics and notation by types of function

FUNCTION TYPE		FUNCTION CONTENT	FUNCTION INDICATION
Function of disease risk reduction		Food intake reduces the risk of disease or health	Helps to reduce the risk of OO occurrence
Physiological function	Physiological function class1	Has a special effect on the normal functioning or biological activity of the human body, indicating a contribution to health, functional improvement, or health maintenance and improvement	Help OO
	Physiological function class2		Can help OO
Nutrient function		Physiological action of nutrients on the normal functioning or biological activity of the human body	

To date, calcium and vitamin D have been shown to help reduce osteoporosis, and xylitol has been shown to help reduce tooth decay. When it corresponds to the disease risk reduction function, it is labeled as "helping to reduce the risk of disease occurrence"; for example, calcium is displayed as "helping to reduce the risk of osteoporosis." Most of the products found in the dietary supplement market belong to bioactive functions that help maintain or improve health. Depending on how it helps the body, it is classified as 31 kinds of functionalities. It can be divided into intestinal health, blood sugar control, and joint/bone health. Each type of functionality and its functional ingredients can be found on the Food Safety Information Portal and the Ministry of Food and Drug Safety. Bioactive functions are classified into two classes according to the scientific basis of product efficacy, and the labeling method is different accordingly. In the case of grades 1 and 2, the clinical trials verify the actual effects on the human body and indicate "help for 00" or "Can help for 00." Nutrient function corresponds to the function of the physiological action of nutrients such as vitamins, minerals, and protein fiber.

Only dietary ingredients that have been validated by the KFDA (MFDS: Ministry of Food and Drug Safety) can be used in dietary supplements. Ingredients can be divided into two types according to their characteristics, which are classified into "Notified Ingredients," which are the Director of the Ministry of Food and Drugs published standards and specifications in the Health Functional Korean Food Standards Codex, and "Individually Certified Ingredients," which have been approved by the Director of the KFDA (MFDS) (Table 8.3).

The raw materials of the public notice type are registered as the health functional foods after completing the verification of the functions of the raw materials at the health functional food code, so the product can be developed without additional certification procedure. To date, about 95 kinds of raw materials have been listed, and they include tree ear mushroom extract, sang-hwang mushroom extract, and aloe gel. Individually recognized raw materials, on the other hand, are not specified in the dietary supplement, but are separately approved by the health functional food code. Only these companies can use the ingredients for dietary supplements, and about 200 functional ingredients are listed. Health functional food aims to maintain a healthy life through maintaining the normal function of the body or physiological function. The proven functionality of health function foods does not directly cure or prevent disease through health function foods, which is different from the efficacy of medicine.

Table 8.3 Characteristics of health functional food's raw material

DIVISION	NOTICE ON TYPE OF RAW MATERIAL	INDIVIDUALLY RECOGNIZED RAW MATERIALS
Main content	• Functional raw material listed in the health functional food standard codex • If the product meets the manufacturing standards, specifications, and requirements of the final product, the product can be produced and sold without additional certification	• Raw material that are individually recognized by the director of the KFDA as functional ingredients not listed in the Health Functional Food standard codex. • Production/sale of products requires review of data on the safety, functionality, standards, and specifications of the raw materials.
Monopolistic rights	None	Manufactured/sold only by certified supplier
Example	Aloe gel, Sichuan mushroom extract	Schisandra fruit extract, pomegranate concentrate powder

Until health functional foods are put on the market, manufacturers are first recognized for the functionality of the raw materials, then process the functional raw materials to produce products, distribute and consume them, and provide them to consumers. The detailed management system for each step is shown in Figure 8.5.

At the stage of functional raw material recognition, manufacturers and importers apply for approval to KFDA based on data on functionality, safety, and criteria/standards to be recognized for the functionality of raw materials. The KFDA reviews and judges the functionality of raw materials in consultation with the Health Functional Food Review Committee. For functional ingredients, the raw material is entered into the production stage, where the manufacturer and importer registers GMP-Good Manufacturing Practice with the KFDA and declares hygiene and quality control. In addition, it is decided how to advertise the product during the production stage. Currently, the KFDA conducts the preliminary deliberation on the functional label advertisement with the label advertisement review committee of the health functional food association. Finally, during the consumption phase of the distribution, the product is monitored for problems. If an abnormal case occurs, the manufacturer, importer, or distributor reports the case to the KFDA.

With the growing interest in healthy food, the dietary supplement market is growing at a very rapid pace. As a result, you can find a variety of dietary supplement products in the market and the first thing to consider when selecting a dietary supplement is to check the health functional food certification mark. Aligned to the Ministry of Food and Drug Safety, only the products that have passed the inspection and whose functionality has been verified can be labeled with the phrase or certification mark provided by the Food and Drug Administration. Therefore, to select the correct dietary supplement, it must be purchased after confirming that the dietary supplement mark distributed by the KFDA is attached (Figure 8.6).

8.4 Health Functional Foods in the World

The global market for dietary supplements is estimated at US $118.1 billion in 2015, with an average annual growth rate of 7.3% (Commercializations Promotion Agency for R&D Outcomes 2016).

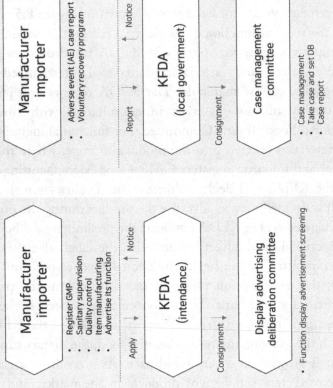

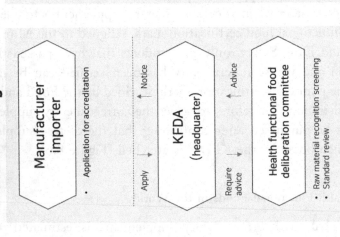

Figure 8.5　Health functional food management system.

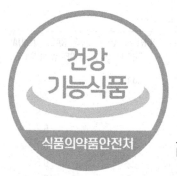

Figure 8.6 Health functional food certification mark.

Based on these statistics, it was projected to reach about $167.7 billion by 2020. The largest share of the world's health functional equipment market is the United States, with a market of about $40.4 billion in 2015 and an average annual growth rate of 7.1%. Then, China which is projected at about $16.3 billion, annual average growth rate of 13.8%, Japan at about US$10.9 billion, and average annual growth rate of 2.3% (Korea Agro-Fisheries & Food Trade Corporation 2016).

The definition of health functional food differs from country to country, and the term "supplements" is the most common term used to refer to health functional food, and some countries include the words functional and health. Health functional foods in Korea are classified as dietary supplements in the United States, EU uses food supplements, ASEAN uses health supplements, China uses health foods, and Japan uses health functional foods (Nutrition Business Journal 2014). On the other hand, the range of health functional foods in each country and related labeling standards are different. In the United States, it is managed by the U.S. FDA and includes a range of dietary supplements containing vitamins, minerals, and dietary ingredients. The EU manages food authorities in each country and defines food supplements as food supplements with the purpose or physiological impact of dietary supplements in the form of capsules, tablets, and liquid ampoules. In Japan, the Consumer Agency separates and manages individual licensed types as specific health foods and standard types as nutrition functional foods. Lastly, the food that is expressed with specific nutritional function from CFDA or the food that is to supplement vitamin, mineral, etc. are defined as nutritional food (Ministry of Food and Drug Safety 2016).

Table 8.4 Size of health functional food market in each country

MILLION DOLLARS	2012	2013	2015	2020E	PORTION OF 2020	AVERAGE ANNUAL GROWTH RATE
United States	32458	34935	40376	56782	34	7.2
West Europe	15909	16193	16837	19033	11	2.3
Japan	10551	10624	10898	12184	7	1.8
Canada	1679	1761	1946	2530	2	5.3
China	11893	13253	16307	26726	16	10.7
Other Asia	9024	9884	11843	18670	22	9.5
Latin America	6275	7092	8928	15532	9	12
Australia/New Zealand	2051	2149	2380	3107	2	5.3
East Europe/ Russia	4490	4952	6006	9423	6	9.7
Middle East/Asia	997	1093	1312	2084	1	9.7
Africa	789	860	1092	1608	1	9.3
Total	96116	102796	117862	167679	100	7.2

Below are the characteristics of the dietary supplement market by country (Table 8.4).

The United States defines health functional food as dietary supplements, making it the largest market in the world. On further analysis, as of 2015, other specialty foods accounted for the highest share of the market at 43.9%, followed by vitamins and minerals at 38.5% (Korea Agro-Fisheries & Food Trade Corporation 2016). Research shows that more than 66% of all Americans had taken vitamins and dietary supplements regularly in 2017 (Carolina Ordonez 2017). This seems to be due to the recent increase in weight, childhood obesity, and adult lifestyle diseases, as well as the aging population and the burden of health insurance premiums. Therefore, the U.S. functional food market is expected to continue to grow as it is today. In particular, the market for other specialty functional foods has grown significantly in recent years. In line with this trend, it is expected that various health functional foods such as children's health functional food, weight control products and products developed for the sports market will be introduced to the market in the future.

China forms the world's second-largest health functional food market. However, unlike in the United States, vitamins and minerals accounted for 42.1%, and herbs and plant extracts accounted for 41.1% (Korea Agro-Fisheries & Food Trade Corporation 2016). In addition, the share of specialty functional foods was the lowest in the United States but lately the demand for health functional food is steadily increasing in China due to rapid economic development. In addition, as China is aging rapidly and young people's interest in health is increasing, the potential of China's health functional food market is expected to develop in the future aligned to these demographic trends. Currently China's health functional food market is mainly about products related to women's beauty, products that help prevent kidney disease and diabetes, and improve sleep. Meanwhile, with the rapid development of the economy, China, like the United States, is introducing various sports nutritional health food products to the market. China's specialty health foods include herbal medicine, Chinese herbal medicine, diet tea, and ginkgo extract. Since Chinese health foods have no restrictions on formulation, it is a distinguishing feature that currently registered products include teas and beverages that are in the form of general foods.

Japan has the world's third-largest market for health functional food. Japan's rapidly aging society is potentially able to support a large dietary supplement market despite its smaller population than the United States or China. However, in Japan, the market growth rate is very slow compared to the market size and the aged population. The Japanese dietary supplement market has grown rapidly until 2007, but it seems to have been stagnant for the past 10 years. This is due to the recent decline in the population in their 30s and 50s, which have the economic power of Japan (Figure 8.7) (Lee and Han 2016). Health functional foods are more selective than essential to life. As a result, the market for health functional food is likely to be driven by consumers who have purchasing power. Looking at the current state of the health functional food market in Japan, the size of the market is determined by the increase in the population in their 30s and 50s. This can also be confirmed by the trend of the Japanese health functional food market, where the health functional food that help beauty and joints are leading the market. As a result, contrary to the expectations of many experts that the elderly population will

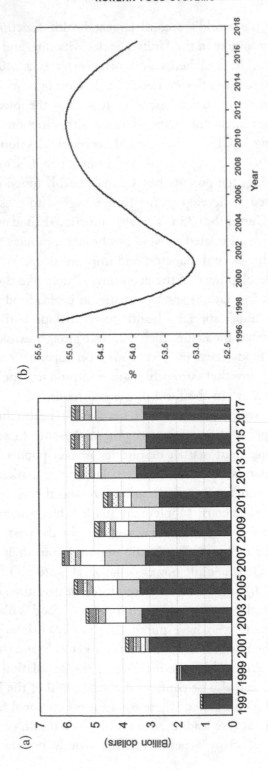

Figure 8.7 Market size of health functional food in Japan and the growth rate of the 30s–50s population.

increase and the dietary supplement market will grow at the same time, the dietary supplement market in Japan has stagnated due to the decline in middle-aged people in their 30s and 50s with purchasing power.

The same is happening in Germany. The stagnation in the health functional food market in Germany is even worse than in Japan. According to the survey, the German health functional food market has declined 6.6% over the last 5 years. This contrasts with a 5% increase in the German elderly population over the last 5 years, while a 1.3% decrease in the population in their 20s and 50s (Han 2016). In other words, Germany, like Japan, suggests that the market for health functional food is determined by middle-aged people who have purchasing power, not elderly people. In the case of Germany and Japan, it is understood that the consumption of health functional food is active even in middle-aged people, whereas the main consumers of health functional food were thought to be the elderly. Overall, the trend of the health functional food market is changing. This phenomenon can be confirmed in the domestic market. As mentioned previously, interest in inner beauty is increasing among women in their 20s and 30s, and the market size is increasing rapidly.

As another example, when looking at the Vietnamese health functional food market as of 2017, the size of the Vietnamese health functional food market is estimated at 20,5928 billion dong. Recently, the Vietnamese health functional food market recorded double-digit growth every year. According to the survey, the annual average growth rate of the Vietnamese health functional food market was 13.1% (Yoon 2018). In short, the market is growing very rapidly. If the Vietnamese market continues to grow, experts predict that after 5 years it will be 40% larger than it is now. This seems to be due to the increased awareness of the health by Vietnamese consumers due to the recent increase in Internet usage. However, more than 70% of the health functional foods in the Vietnamese market are foreign brands, and only a few of them are manufactured and sold by pure Vietnamese companies. The Vietnamese market has recently grown, so it appears that it has not formed a unique domestic brand yet. Recognized products in the Vietnamese market are those from the United States, Europe, and Japan, which are being accepted by consumers due to the recognition that alternative cheaper Chinese products are likely to be of poor quality or counterfeit.

It is no exaggeration to say that the biggest issue and trend of the recent food market is health functional food. In some countries, such as Japan and Germany, the market for health functional food has stagnated, but this is only caused by a decrease in the number of middle-aged populations with purchasing power. On the other hand, in the countries that have recently witnessed rapid economic development, the growth is very large, and the growth and development of the functional food market is expected to increase further in the future.

8.5 The Future of Health Functional Foods

As self-care "self-medication" has recently become a new trend, the number of young consumers purchasing health functional food has increased, the market is steadily expanding, and the consumption pattern types are also changing from "general" to "personalization." The wide variety of raw materials and products' reduced price and easy access has given personalized dietary options new popularity. Health functional foods have also arrived in an age where people can choose and eat products according to their needs such as gender, age, and living environment.

Overall change in the health functional foods market seems to be affected by the gradual decline in the age group of dietary supplement consumers. The middle-aged, mainly consumed functional foods in preparation for a healthy old age, whereas the young consumers who are busy with their daily life, take it for health care. As the purchasing power of young consumers in their 20s and 30s continue to grow, the necessity of diversity and customization for products is needed. In other words, health functional foods in the future are expected to be developed in the form of analyzing the lifestyle of individual consumers and providing products that satisfy the actual necessary nutrients through various diagnostic indicator systems. In line with this, products to improve the absorption rate, bioavailability, and stability of functional raw materials and combining raw materials according to individual needs, the application of nanotechnology and 3D printing technology is expected.

The term *nano* is a Greek word derived from "nanos" and is now used as a physical measurement unit, meaning one out of a billion (Kim et al. 2014). Nanotechnology is a cutting-edge technology that operates up to 1 billionth of a meter and can be applied to various technologies in the food field. It is evaluated as the next-generation core technology that can improve quality of human health and overall life with the ability to solve existing problems of the food industry. Nanotechnology has been the center of development of new manufacturing industry based on advanced manufacturing technology along with information technology and biotechnology. Since early 2000, many efforts have been made for industrialization and research in various countries in these advanced research domains.

Many health-targeted functional substances are limited in physiological activity due to their stability to the external environment and their low solubility during digestion and absorption, which means that only a very small amount is used *in vivo* compared to the amount consumed. For example, red ginseng, one of Korea's favorite health functional foods, is known as a major physiologically active substance, but in fact, 37.5% of Koreans lack the ability to decompose and absorb saponin (Ham et al. 2004). Also, curcumin, which is commonly extracted from turmeric and known as a curry ingredient, is a recognized dietary supplement, but its body absorption rate is less than 1% (Park and Ahn 2015). The activity may decrease even more due to several factors such as temperature, oxygen, light, etc. during processing and storage of dietary supplements. Encapsulating the functional material using food nanotechnology can increase the utilization rate in the body and protect it from external factors such as temperature, oxygen, and water. It also helps reach the right targets in the body when it is most efficient without any degradation of functional ingredients such as vitamins. These strategies can control the release rate to maintain optimal concentration in the body or also be used as a tissue-specific target delivery system. Like the Korean saying, "beads are only useful when they are braided." Functional foods even with the best ingredients are useless if the absorption rate is low. It is expected that health functional foods with a high absorption rate will become the new trend (Figure 8.8).

"Personalized medicine" provides services tailored to the individual's health characteristics, and is one of the major trends

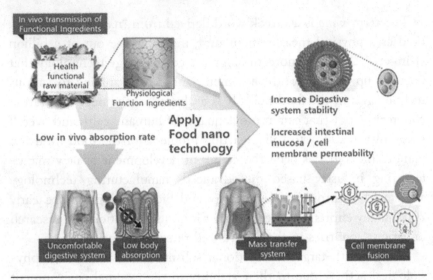

Figure 8.8   Improved absorption rate of functional raw materials using food nanotechnology.

leading the healthcare industry in recent years. The dietary supplement market is no exception to this trend, and it is expected to evolve in the form of prescribing, combining, and supplying products that meet the nutritional needs of individuals. In the field of nutritional genomics in the healthcare industry, the influence of certain nutrients and functional components on genes have been identified. To provide customized components consistent with this genetic profile, investments are being made to introduce genomics, big data, and 3D printing technologies to personalized manufacturing technologies, which are attracting attention for the Fourth Industrial Revolution. Most notable among them is 3D food printing technology, which can be used to design personalized dietary supplements that are close to ideal for delivering functional benefits (Park and Kim 2018).

3D food printing technology is a digital manufacturing technology that reconstructs food in three-dimensional form by stacking foods based on three-dimensional modeling data generated by CAD or 3D scanners. This is used as baseline technology for small quantity batch production that can meet individual needs beyond the limitations of the existing large scale functional food production system. The materials used for 3D printing are supplied in the form of powder or dough, and in these formulations functional materials manufactured

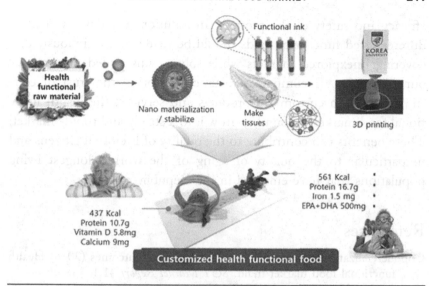

Figure 8.9 Production of personalized dietary supplement food using 3D printing technology.

by nanotechnology can be easily incorporated. This enables precise control of components for individuals while improving the absorption and bioavailability of functional raw materials (Figure 8.9).

Today, 3D food printing technology has reached a level where you can program food to suit your nutritional needs, as well as the appearance of food. Due to the open source of design data, existing production methods have shifted to digital domains, accelerating production strategies and movement to wider applications. As the technology evolves and the price of equipment decreases, it is expected to become a new strategic solution application in the manufacture of personalized dietary supplements.

As seen by the trends, the growth of the health functional food market is expected to continue. However, consumers are often hesitant to purchase due to high price or uncertainty about efficacy. Korea has already established and improved various regulations on health functional foods through the "Health Functional Food Law." As a result, some of the practices introduced as panacea have disappeared to some extent. However, the technology level and the characteristics of products among health functional food manufacturers vary widely. For this reason, it is not easy to improve the awareness of health functional foods. Above all, it is time to clearly show evidence of functionality of the main ingredients to prove the efficacy and safety of the product. In addition, the development of differentiated functional foods should be made by continuously discovering unexplored markets while solving unsatisfied demands of our consumers. If companies focus on restoring the trust of consumers through customized products and services, the health functional food market is bound to grow into a steady and trendy market. These benefits can contribute to the quality of life of all citizens and in particular to the quality of aging of the world's longest living populations that have emerged in the Republic of Korea.

References

Commercializations Promotion Agency for R&D Outcomes (2016) Health functional food market trend. *S&T Market Report* 41:1–34.

Euromonitor International (2017) Vitamins and Dietary Supplements (VDS): Trends and Prospects 2017.

Ham SH, Kim HJ, Kim MJ, Park YG, Kim JB (2004) A study on the individual difference of Ginseng saponin degradation by intestinal microorganisms in Koreans. *The Korean Society of Food Science and Nutrition* 11:17–19.

Han JA (2016) "[Health food market analyis1] Market stagnation due to aging…'30~50s are the leading players'". *FETV*. https://www.fetv.co.kr/news/article.html?no=2487

Iwatani S, and Yamamoto N (2019) Functional food products in Japan: A review. *Food Science and Human Wellness* 8(2):96–101.

Kim GS, Choi DJ, Lee SH, Lee DY, Park CG, Kim HD, Park CH and Ahn YS (2016) The healthy food which has functional specialty. *RDA Interrobang* 181:1–29.

Kim SH, Kim BS and Ko SH (2014) Nanotechnology-applied food: Definition and application category. *Food Science and Industry* 47(1):2–11.

Korea Agro-Fisheries & Food Trade Corporation (2016) 2016 Processed food segment market status-Health functional foods. 50–56.

Korea Health Supplements Association (2017) Health functional food market status and consumer survey report 2017. 60–88.

Lee HJ and Han KH (2016) Nutribiotech-A leap to becoming a global ODM health functional food company. *NH Investment & Securities*:1–44.

Legal text on functional health foods (2018.6.12. Law No. 15706).

Ministry of food and drug safety (2016) Strategy seminar for global health functional food development material.

Nutrition Business Journal (2014) NBJ's Global Supplement and Nutrition Industry Report 2014: An analysis of markets, trends, competition, and strategy in the Global Nutrition Industry. 241–288.

Park HJ and Ahn YJ (2015) Absorption Improvement of curcumin powder using Theracurmin®. *Food Science Industry* 48(2):42–46.

Park HJ and Kim HW (2018) The future of 3D food printing and the food industry. *2018 Nation Nutrition* 41:42–46.

Park SH (2012) A study on the classification and utilization of 100 Korean commercial foods by 氣味論 (theory of taste energy) according to efficacy. *Yulchon Foundation Food Related Basic Research Papers* 4:793–989.

Regulations on the functional ingredients and functional standards (2016.12.21. Ministry of food and drug safety notice No. 2016-141).

Weststrate JA, Van Poppel G and Verschuren PM (2002) Functional foods, trends, and future. *British Journal of Nutrition* 88(S2):S233–S235.

Yoon BN (2018) Diverse demand for health functional foods in Vietnam. *Kotra Overseas Market News*.

Index

NOTE: Italics indicates a figure; boldface indicates a table.

Printed in the United States
by Baker & Taylor Publisher Services